MOLECULAR
BIOLOGY
INTELLIGENCE
UNIT

THE HUMAN T-CELL RECEPTOR REPERTOIRE AND TRANSPLANTATION

Peter J. van den Elsen, Ph.D.

Department of Immunohematology and Blood Bank
University Hospital Leiden
Leiden, The Netherlands

Springer-Verlag Berlin Heidelberg GmbH

R.G. LANDES COMPANY
AUSTIN

MOLECULAR BIOLOGY INTELLIGENCE UNIT

THE HUMAN T-CELL RECEPTOR REPERTOIRE AND TRANSPLANTATION

R.G. LANDES COMPANY
Austin, Texas, U.S.A.

Submitted: May 1995
Published: July 1995

International Copyright © 1995 Springer-Verlag Berlin Heidelberg
Originally published by Springer-Verlag, Heidelberg, Germany in 1995
Softcover reprint of the hardcover 1st edition 1995

All rights reserved.

International ISBN 978-3-662-22496-0

While the authors, editors and publisher believe that drug selection and dosage and the specifications and usage of equipment and devices, as set forth in this book, are in accord with current recommendations and practice at the time of publication, they make no warranty, expressed or implied, with respect to material described in this book. In view of the ongoing research, equipment development, changes in governmental regulations and the rapid accumulation of information relating to the biomedical sciences, the reader is urged to carefully review and evaluate the information provided herein.

Library of Congress Cataloging-in-Publicatiuon Data

Van den Elsen, Peter J., 1951-
The human T-cell receptor repertoire and transplantation / by Peter J. van den Elsen
p. cm. — (Molecular biology intelligence unit)
Includes bibliographical reference and index.
ISBN 978-3-662-22496-0 ISBN 978-3-662-22494-6 (eBook)
DOI 10.1007/978-3-662-22494-6
1. Graft rejection. 2. T-cells—Receptors. 3. Transplantation immunology. I. Title. II. Series.
[DNLM: 1. Receptors, Antigen, T-Cell—immunology. 2. Graft Rejection—immunology. 3. T-lymphocytes—immunology. QW 573 V227h 1995]
QR188.8.V36 1995
616.07'9—dc20
DNLM/DNLC
for Library of Congress 95-14122
CIP

Publisher's Note

R.G. Landes Company publishes five book series: *Medical Intelligence Unit, Molecular Biology Intelligence Unit, Neuroscience Intelligence Unit, Tissue Engineering Intelligence Unit* and *Biotechnology Intelligence Unit*. The authors of our books are acknowledged leaders in their fields and the topics are unique. Almost without exception, no other similar books exist on these topics.

Our goal is to publish books in important and rapidly changing areas of medicine for sophisticated researchers and clinicians. To achieve this goal, we have accelerated our publishing program to conform to the fast pace in which information grows in biomedical science. Most of our books are published within 90 to 120 days of receipt of the manuscript. We would like to thank our readers for their continuing interest and welcome any comments or suggestions they may have for future books.

Deborah Muir Molsberry
Publications Director
R.G. Landes Company

CONTENTS

===== EDITOR =====

Peter J. van den Elsen
Department of Immunohematology and Blood Bank
University Hospital Leiden
Leiden, The Netherlands
Chapters 1-8

===== CONTRIBUTORS =====

David M. Andrews
Department of Pathology
Massachusetts General Hospital
Boston, Massachusetts, U.S.A.
Chapter 4

Carla Baan
Department of Internal Medicine
University Hospital Dykzigt-
  Rotterdam
Rotterdam, The Netherlands
Chapter 6

Lenora A. Boyle
Department of Pathology
Massachusetts General Hospital
Boston, Massachusetts, U.S.A.
Chapter 4

Jan Antony Bruijn
Department of Pathology
University Hospital Leiden
Leiden, The Netherlands
Chapters 5, 7

Frans J. Claas
Department of Immunohematology
  and Blood Bank
University Hospital Leiden
Leiden, The Netherlands
Chapters 6, 7

Rene Daane
Department of Internal Medicine
University Hospital Dykzigt-
  Rotterdam
Rotterdam, The Netherlands
Chapter 6

Mohamed R. Daha
Department of Nephrology
University Hospital Leiden
Leiden, The Netherlands
Chapters 5, 7

Gert Datema
Department of Immunohematology
  and Blood Bank
University Hospital Leiden
Leiden, The Netherlands
Chapter 6

Marja van Eggermond
Department of Immunohematology
  and Blood Bank
University Hospital Leiden
Leiden, The Netherlands
Chapter 2

CONTRIBUTORS

Leendert A. van Es
Department of Nephrology
University Hospital Leiden
Leiden, The Netherlands
Chapters 5, 7

Barbara Godthelp
Department of Immunohematology
   and Blood Bank
University Hospital Leiden
Leiden, The Netherlands
Chapter 2

Gail E. Hawes
Department of Immunohematology
   and Blood Bank
University Hospital Leiden
Leiden, The Netherlands
Chapters 2, 3

Makiko Kumagai-Braesch
Department of Pathology
Massachusetts General Hospital
Boston, Massachusetts, U.S.A.
Chapter 4

James T. Kurnick
Department of Pathology
Massachusetts General Hospital
Boston, Massachusetts, U.S.A.
Chapter 4

Carol P. Leary
Department of Pathology
Massachusetts General Hospital
Boston, Massachusetts, U.S.A.
Chapter 4

M.E. Paape
Department of Nephrology
University Hospital Leiden
Leiden, The Netherlands
Chapter 5

Frank Raaphorst
Department of Immunohematology
   and Blood Bank
University Hospital Leiden
Leiden, The Netherlands
Chapter 2

Thomas Reterink
Department of Immunohematology
   and Blood Bank
University Hospital Leiden
Leiden, The Netherlands
Chapters 5, 7

Linda Struyk
Department of Immunohematology
   and Blood Bank
University Hospital Leiden
Leiden, The Netherlands
Chapter 2

Richard Waitkus
Department of Pathology
Massachusetts General Hospital
Boston, Massachusetts, U.S.A.
Chapter 4

Willem Weimar
Department of Internal Medicine
University Hospital Dykzigt-
   Rotterdam
Rotterdam, The Netherlands
Chapter 6

CONTRIBUTORS

Len Vaessen
Department of Internal Medicine
University Hospital Dykzigt-
  Rotterdam
Rotterdam, The Netherlands
Chapter 6

Fokko J. van der Woude
Department of Nephrology
University Hospital Leiden
Leiden, The Netherlands
Chapters 5, 7

Benito A. Yard
Department of Nephrology
University Hospital Leiden
Leiden, The Netherlands
Chapters 5, 7

ACKNOWLEDGMENTS

I would like to thank the publishers of Human Immunology, the Journal of Immunology, International Immunology, Immunogenetics, Kidney International and Transplantation for granting permission to use some of the figures and tables presented in chapters 2, 5 and 6 which were previously published in these journals. Special thanks also to my other collaborators Jeroen van Bergen, Jan Bruining, Eric Kaijzel, Maarten van der Keur, Ronald de Krijger, Renee Langlois-van den Berg, Maarten van Tol and Jaak Vossen for their contributions and support, Sam Gobin for his art-work and Karin Vlasveld for endless editing sessions of the manuscripts presented in this overview.

======= CHAPTER 1 =======

GENERAL INTRODUCTION

Peter J. van den Elsen

1. INTRODUCTION

This book presents a number of studies concerning the human T-cell receptor (TCR) repertoire and transplantation. In transplantation, the major complication is acute cellular rejection. The immunological mechanisms that mediate allograft rejection are not yet fully understood but it is well established that T-lymphocytes play an important role through recognition of peptide antigens presented in the context of major histocompatibility complex (MHC) molecules expressed by the allograft. These complexes of MHC and peptide are seen as foreign by the immune repertoire of the host. The function of MHC class I molecules is to present peptides which originate from endogenous sources whereas MHC class II molecules present mainly peptides that originate from the exogenous antigen processing pathway. These complexes of MHC and peptide serve as ligands for the αβ T-cell receptor of cytotoxic T cells (MHC class I) or helper T cells (MHC class II). Both MHC class I and class II molecules are extremely polymorphic, and each allelic form can present a specific subset of peptides. T-cell recognition of antigens requires that they are processed into peptides and that these peptide antigens subsequently are presented by MHC class I or class II molecules at the surface of an antigen presenting cell (APC). Formation of a trimolecular complex of MHC, peptide and TCR is a prerequisite for T-cell activation prior to exertion of T-cell function, explaining the phenomenon of MHC restriction of antigen recognition.

During T-cell development in the thymus various complexes of MHC and peptide expressed in the thymic microenvironment play a pivotal role in the shaping of the T-cell repertoire. As a result, the peripheral T-cell repertoire is non-responsive to the subset of self peptides presented by autologous MHC alleles, but is responsive to complexes of

The Human T-Cell Receptor Repertoire and Transplantation, edited by Peter J. van den Elsen. © 1995 R.G. Landes Company.

allo MHC and peptide. Consequently, alloreactive T-lymphocytes play a major role in graft rejection in transplantation.

A brief overview will be given of the results of the current state of MHC research, T-cell development and models for allo recognition. Furthermore, various approaches for studying the T-cell receptor repertoire will be discussed.

1.1 THE STRUCTURE OF MHC CLASS I AND CLASS II MOLECULES

The human major histocompatibility complex (MHC) is located on the short arm of chromosome 6 in the distal part of the 6p21.3 band and spans about 4Mb. Its gene products are predominantly associated with the immune system.[1] MHC class I and class II molecules play a pivotal role in the host defense mechanism against foreign pathogens by virtue of their ability to present peptide antigens to T lymphocytes. The classical MHC class I molecules are encoded by three different genes called HLA-A, B and C. The products of these genes are expressed as integral membrane proteins on almost all nucleated cells in association with β_2-microglobulin. More recently a number of additional genes have been described which share great sequence homology with the HLA-A, B and C genes. These so called MHC class I-like genes, which include HLA-E, F and G, have a different tissue-distribution when compared to classical MHC class I genes.[2,3]

The classical MHC class II molecules comprise the HLA-DR, DQ and DP antigens. They are integral membrane proteins consisting of an α and a β chain each of which is encoded by different genes. In contrast to class I MHC molecules, the MHC class II antigens are expressed primarily by specialized antigen presenting cells such as macrophages, dendritic cells and B-lymphocytes.

MHC class I molecules are glycoproteins with an approximate size of 44 kD. The class I molecule consist of an extracellular portion which is comprised of three domains (α_1, α_2 and α_3), a transmembrane region (TM) and a cytoplasmic tail (CT). These various functional domains which can be distinguished, are each encoded by different exons within the gene. One of the hallmarks of the classical MHC class I antigens is their great polymorphism within the general outbred population. Currently at least 50 different HLA-A, 97 different HLA-B and 34 different HLA-C alleles can be distinguished.[4] This has been determined both by serological and DNA-typing. When expressed on the cell membrane, the HLA class I molecule is associated with β_2-microglobulin. This latter molecule is non-polymorphic, has a molecular weight of 12 kD and does not penetrate the cell membrane. Association of β_2-microglobulin with the MHC class I molecule occurs through interaction with amino acids present within the MHC class I encoded α_3 domain.

From X-ray diffraction analysis of crystals, the structure of MHC class I molecules HLA-A2, Aw68 and B27 has been elucidated.[5-8] From these analyses it became clear that the MHC class I molecule comprised a distinct groove on the external side of the molecule. The sides of the groove are formed by the α-helical structures of the $α_1$ and $α_2$ domains and a floor which is formed by 8 anti-parallel β strands. The various polymorphic residues, as determined from DNA sequence analysis, are localized within these α-helices and β-plated sheets within the groove. More importantly, these analyses also revealed the presence of electron-dense material in the groove. This material was subsequently identified as a linear peptide of 8-10 amino acids long.[5,6,8-10] High resolution crystallographic analyses of the class I MHC structure have revealed the existence of so-called pockets within the grooves of the MHC class I molecules. These pockets designated A-F, exhibited allele-specificity and are directly involved in the binding of the peptide, primarily through interaction with the dominant anchor residues as found in MHC class I associated peptides.[6,7,9,11]

The class II MHC antigens consist on the cell surface of a 34 kD α chain non-covalently associated with a 28 kD β chain. With the exception of the DR α-chain, all other MHC class II α and β chains are polymorphic. Recently, the crystal structure of the MHC class II molecule (HLA-DR1) has been resolved.[12] Both the α and β chains of HLA-DR1 contribute to the formation of an externally faced groove which is in essence similarly structured as the MHC class I groove. Similar to MHC class I molecules, pockets can be found within the class II MHC grooves that are involved in peptide binding.[13] In contrast to MHC class I molecules, the groove of MHC class II was found to contain peptides of longer length, usually consisting of 13-26 amino acids.

A schematic representation of MHC class I and class II molecules is depicted in Figure 1.1. Both in MHC class I and class II molecules nearly all the polymorphic amino acid residues are located at the antigen binding site, accounting for the differential ability of different allelic forms to bind a variety of different peptides.

1.2 ORIGIN AND STRUCTURE OF PEPTIDES ASSOCIATED WITH MHC CLASS I AND II MOLECULES

MHC class I associated peptides

MHC class I molecules in general present peptides which originate from endogenous sources. These peptides can be derived from the degradation of normal cellular proteins, from proteins encoded by foreign pathogens expressed by cells that have been infected or from proteins which are expressed de novo following cellular transformation. It is estimated that on normal cells over 10,000 different peptides can be found to be associated with MHC class I molecules expressed on the cell membrane.[14] Of these, approximately 2000 distinct peptides are relatively abundantly present in the grooves of the expressed MHC class I molecules.[15,16]

In humans, the predominant length of peptides associated with most MHC class I molecules is nine amino acid residues,[10,15,17-21] although longer peptides have also been identified which can bind to MHC class I molecules with affinities comparable to those of the predominant forms.[22]

Pool sequencing by Edman degradation of unfractionated peptide mixtures has revealed the presence of dominant amino acid residues.[23-27] These so-called "anchor" residues play an important role in the binding properties of the peptide to the MHC class I molecules. In particular the carboxy-terminal amino acid residue of the peptide is crucial for binding to MHC class I molecules by virtue of its ability to interact with the F-pocket of the peptide-binding groove of the MHC class I antigen. In a similar fashion, the conserved amino acid residue usually found at position 2 or 5 of MHC class I associated peptides respectively interacts with the B- or C-pockets of the MHC class I peptide-binding groove. Recently, the significance of the six peptide-binding pockets of HLA-A2.1 for peptide binding and subsequent cytotoxic T cell (CTL) recognition was investigated. Influenza A matrix peptide-specific cytotoxic T-lymphocyte reactivity was evaluated taking advantage of a library of mutated HLA-A2.1 molecules with amino acid substitutions in all six peptide binding pockets.[28,29] Mutations in the B-pocket significantly affected the influenza A-matrix peptide 58-66 specific CTL recognition suggesting that the B-pocket plays a crucial role in the CTL recognition of this peptide. However, mutations in

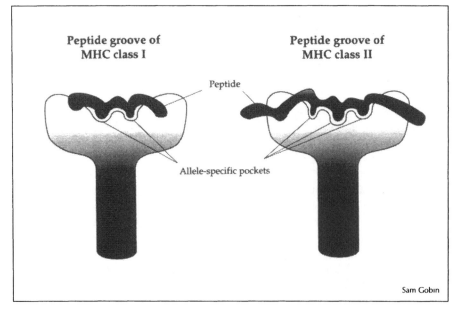

Fig. 1.1. Schematic representation of MHC class I and class II antigens and associated peptide.

all other HLA-A2.1 pockets, except for pocket F, also affected CTL recognition. These observations suggest that in addition to the pockets critical for peptide binding, the pockets which play a less pronounced role in peptide binding, are crucial for influenza A matrix peptide 58-66 specific CTL recognition.

Among the naturally processed antigens expressed by normal cells, peptides derived from MHC molecules can be found.[20,30] In this respect among the peptide pools eluted from HLA-A2.1 and HLA-B7 peptides derived from the signal sequences of class I(-like) molecules HLA A2.1, B7 and E and the class II HLA-DP molecule have been identified.[15,17] These peptides, derived from signal sequences of membrane bound proteins, are generated through the second pathway for antigen processing and presentation[12,31,32] and are capable of eliciting a T cell mediated immune response.[33] The identification of HLA derived peptides among the peptide pools eluted from MHC class I molecules suggest that they play a role in the shaping of the T-cell receptor repertoire in vivo.

MHC class II associated peptides

MHC class II molecules present peptides that originate from the exogenous antigen processing pathway. Most of the MHC class II associated peptides that have been identified to date are derived from cellular proteins. Peptides from plasma membrane proteins are frequently found among MHC class II associated peptides. Of interest is the finding that peptides derived from MHC related molecules predominate in the pool of naturally processed peptides presented by MHC class II molecules.[20,34,35] In contrast to human MHC class I associated peptides, the size of which in general is confined to 9 amino acids, peptides binding to MHC class II molecules are longer and more variable in length.[34,35] On average, they comprise between 14 and 18 amino acids in length, but peptides as long as 24 amino acids have been isolated from human MHC class II molecules.[34,36,37] A striking feature of MHC class II molecules is that they can present the same core region of the peptide in a set of peptides that are truncated at their amino and carboxy termini.[35,37] Furthermore, MHC class II associated peptides can extrude the peptide-binding groove both at the amino- and carboxy-terminal sites.

When compared to MHC class I associated peptides, the identification of so-called "anchor residues" is much more difficult but several binding motifs have been deduced in various studies which included binding experiments using synthetic peptide analogs, M13 display libraries and pool sequencing of naturally occurring peptides.[38-42] In contrast to MHC class I binding peptides which exhibit allele specificity, peptides binding to MHC class II molecules have been identified which can associate with almost all class II alleles. Examples of these so-called promiscuous peptides are peptides derived from the invariant chain, HLA-class I (A2-like) and teta-nus toxoid.[35-37,41,43-46]

1.3 ANTIGEN PROCESSING AND PRESENTATION

MHC class I

Peptides presented by MHC class I molecules are derived from endogenously synthesized proteins. They are generated in the cytosol presumably through the action of proteasomes and, in addition, peptidases (Fig. 1.2). It should be noted, however, that the recently identified proteasome related LMP genes which are localized within the MHC do not seem to play a direct role in antigen degradation since they are not essential for antigen presentation by MHC class I.[47,48] These cytosolic peptides must enter the endoplasmic reticulum (ER) to interact with the luminal binding domain of the MHC class I molecule. The products of the TAP1 and TAP2 genes form a heterodimeric structure with twelve transmembrane domains and two ATP binding sites, that resides in the membrane of the ER.[49-52] This complex forms a peptide transporter allowing cytosolic peptides to cross the ER-membrane into the lumen where they are available for coassembly with the newly synthesized MHC class I heavy chain and β2-m. This coassembly in the lumen is aided by accessory molecules like calnexin (p88) since incompletely assembled MHC class I molecules can be found associated with the calnexin (p88) chaperonin. This suggests that dissociation of the calnexin molecule is thought to require both peptide and β2-m to bind to the MHC class I molecule.[53,54] Calnexin is thought to retain in the ER incorrectly assembled MHC class I molecules or to assist in the folding of MHC class I/β2-m complex during biosynthesis. Binding of peptide to the MHC class I/β2-m complex, resulting in dissociation from calnexin, releases the trimolecular complex of MHC class I - peptide -β2-m from its retaining in the ER. This complex is subsequently transported to the cell surface via the network formed by the cis and trans Golgi-apparatus. Stably integrated in the cell membrane of antigen presenting cells, the trimolecular complex of MHC class I - peptide - β2-m can be seen by the clonotypic antigen specific receptors of T cells (the T-cell receptor).

MHC class II

MHC class II molecules are specialized in the presentation of peptides that are generated from exogenous antigens, which are captured by antigen presenting cells (APC) and, following internalization by endocytosis, are processed in the endocytic pathway. In contrast to class I MHC molecules, class II MHC molecules predominantly present peptides derived from proteins occurring in, or directed to, the endosomal/lysosomal compartment of the cell. MHC class II molecules are assembled in the ER by association of an α and β chain, and the

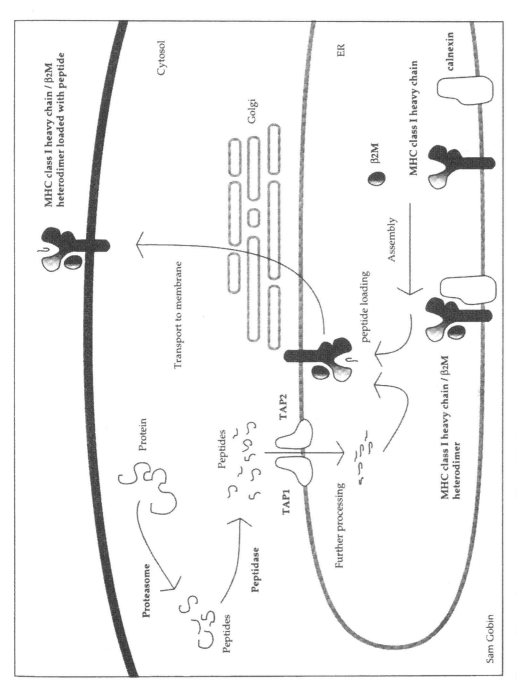

Fig. 1.2. Schematic representation of the MHC class I antigen processing and assembly pathway.

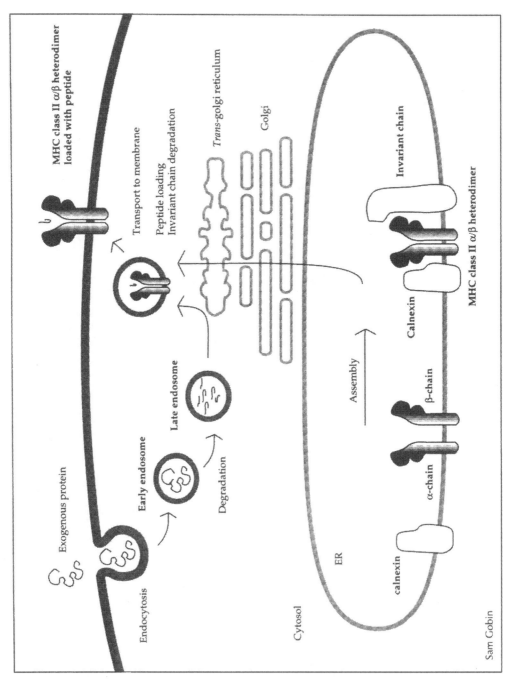

Fig. 1.3. Schematic representation of the MHC class II antigen processing and assembly pathway.

invariant chain (Fig. 1.3). This complex subsequently assembles in the ER into a nonameric structure comprising three α β dimers and the invariant chain trimer. Calnexin (p88) plays an important role in this process by retaining and stabilizing both free class II MHC subunits and partially assembled class II-invariant chain complexes until assembly of the nonamer is complete.[55,56] In the ER binding of peptides from the same pool of peptides that binds to MHC class I molecules is prevented by the invariant chain.[57-59] Binding of the invariant chain to the αβ MHC class II heterodimer induces transport of class II MHC molecules from the ER.[60,61] When formation of the nonamer is complete, calnexin is released from this complex and the MHC/invariant chain nonamer complex is released from the ER. The nonameric complex of the MHC class II αβ chains and invariant chain are further transported through the trans-Golgi reticulum. Here, they are sorted to the endocytic route where the MHC class II molecules will contact internalized and degraded proteins.[62] This sorting is governed by the invariant chain.[63-65] Class II MHC molecules have been observed in early and/or late endosomes[66] as well as lysosomes.[67] However, there are several lines of evidence which suggest that the site of generation of presentable antigen for class II MHC molecules is the lysosome.[67-69] Taken together, these data suggest that the lysosome plays a pivotal role in the generation of peptides as well as peptide loading of class II MHC molecules. In the endocytic pathway the invariant chain is degraded by proteases resulting in restoration of peptide binding capacity of class II MHC molecules.[69,70] MHC class II molecules are transported from the endosomal pathway to the cell surface after release of the invariant chain. At the cell membrane they can present peptides to mainly the CD4 positive subset of T. lymphocytes.

1.4 THE T-CELL RECEPTOR

T-cell recognition of antigens, presented as short peptides by MHC molecules, occurs through the T-cell receptor (TCR), a heterodimeric clonotypic surface molecule usually consisting of an α and β chain (Fig. 1.4). The TCR specificity resides in the variable domains of the α and the β chains of the receptor that are generated during maturation by recombination through somatic rearrangement of germline encoded TCRV (variable), TCRD (diversity, β chain only) and TCRJ (joining) gene segments. In humans, selection from the pool of these TCRV, TCRD and TCRJ region genes allows the potential expression of approximately 10^{15} different TCRs. During recombination, further diversity is generated by mechanisms operating on the TCRAV-TCRAJ and TCRBV-TCRBD-TCRBJ junctions, such as the insertion of non-germline encoded template independent nucleotides (N-nucleotides) or template dependent nucleotides (P-nucleotides). Similar to immunoglobulins, segments of hypervariability can be discerned within TCRV-regions. These so-called complementarity

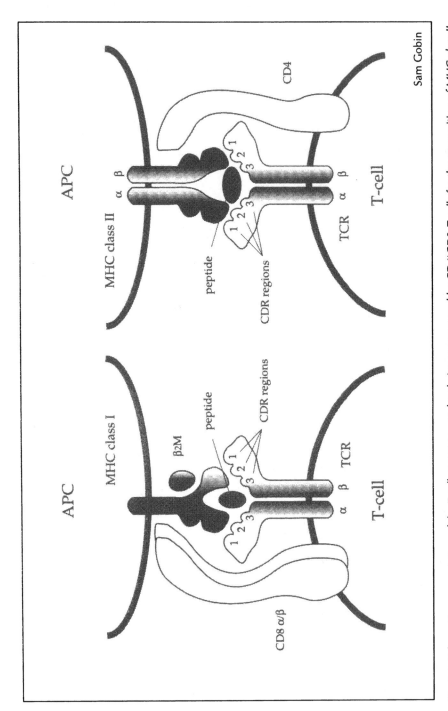

Sam Gobin

Fig. 1.4. Schematic representation of the T-cell receptor α and β chains as expressed by CD4⁺CD8⁻ T cells for the recognition of MHC class II associated peptides and by CD4⁻CD8⁺ T cells for the recognition of MHC class I associated peptides. The regions marked with 1, 2 and 3 represent the CDR1, CDR2 and CDR3 regions of the TCR which are the key elements in the recognition of peptides presented by the MHC.

determining regions (CDR1, 2 and 3) form the antigen binding site. In particular, the CDR3 regions that are the direct products of TCRAV-TCRAJ and TCRBV-TCRBD-TCRBJ joinings make up the central portion of the antigen binding site by directly interacting with the peptide in the groove of the MHC containing, as has emerged from computer modeling studies.[71-73]

The diversity of TCRs is generated in part through the usage of different TCRAV and TCRBV gene segments. This TCRV gene segment usage, however, is not random but is influenced by the genetic background, including the MHC, as has been shown in mice and humans[74-82] in both the CD4$^+$CD8$^-$ and CD4$^-$CD8$^+$ subsets of T lymphocytes.[79,82-87] In addition, usage of TCRBJ segments is biased to either one of these subsets of T lymphocytes as has been shown in mice.[88] In humans, this biased usage of TCRJ segments in T-cell subsets is less pronounced,[89] but in both subsets there is a non-random usage of TCRBJ elements. In particular TCRBJ2S1 and 2S7 are preferentially employed as shown in a number of studies.[89-92] Furthermore, within a given TCRV-gene family, the usage of the individual family-members is non-random.[91] Also of interest is the observation that the nucleotide composition of the CDR3 region is under developmental control.[91,93,94] This has been deduced from the observation that early in fetal development, limited N-region nucleotide additions were found in fetal organs, whereas in later stages of fetal life the number of N-region nucleotides increases suggesting a maturation process in the formation of the antigen binding site. Furthermore, a biased amino-acid composition of the T-cell receptor regions potentially involved in the binding of peptide/MHC complexes is found.[91,95] Taken together, these observations suggest that in normal T-cell development the diversity of the T-cell receptor repertoire is compressed as a consequence of the non-random usage of the various gene elements in TCR β-chain rearrangements and the usage profiles of amino acids in the CDR3 regions.

The actual peripheral T-cell repertoire is a partial representation of the potential repertoire. This is the direct consequence of positive and negative selection events which occur within the thymic micro-environment during T-cell development. These various processes contribute to the generation of the mature peripheral T-cell compartment.[96-100] It is now generally accepted that CD4CD8 double negative (CD4$^-$CD8$^-$) immature T cells enter the thymic differentiation pathway following rearrangement and expression of the TCR β locus. Recent studies, including investigations with transgenic and knock-out mice, have indicated that expression of a TCR β chain, which is not associated with the classical TCR α chain, is pivotal for further differentiation, i.e. acquisition of the CD4CD8 double positive (CD4$^+$CD8$^+$) phenotype and expansion of these thymocytes which express at that stage low numbers of αβ T-cell receptors.[101] The TCR β chain expressed by immature T cells is disulphide linked to a 33 kD glycoprotein and associated in a non-covalent fashion to the components of the CD3 protein ensemble.[102-104] Subsequent interactions of the T-cell receptor (TCR) expressed by these double positive thymocytes and MHC class I or class II antigens expressed by specialized cells within the thymic micro-environment play a crucial role in the negative and positive selection processes.[105,106] Lineage commitment of immature CD4+CD8+ thymocytes is dependent on the avidity of a given TCR, expressed on double positive thymocytes, for MHC class I or class II antigens. In this instructive model TCR-MHC class I or II interactions dictate the resulting single positive phenotype (CD4-CD8+ or CD4+CD8-, respectively) of the mature T cell through down-modulation of the CD4 or CD8 co-receptor.[107,108] As a result, only T cells bearing TCRs with appropriate affinity for "self" MHC class I or class II can be found in the periphery.[109,110] However, the specificity of TCRs for MHC class I or II antigens can be influenced in part by the coexpressed accessory molecules (CD8 or CD4, respectively).[111,112]

Interference in the interactions involved in this selection process has a dramatic effect on the composition of the peripheral T-cell compartment. This has been elegantly demonstrated in the mouse where disturbance of the TCR/MHC class II or class I antigen interaction in neonates due to masking of I-A antigens with anti-class II or H-2 antigens with anti-K^s/D^s monoclonal antibodies resulted in diminished numbers of peripheral CD4+CD8- or CD4-CD8+ T cells respectively.[113-115] Similarly, mice that lack MHC class II expression have greatly reduced numbers of CD4+CD8- peripheral T cells[116,117] whereas mice that lack class I heavy chain expression due to a disrupted β2-microglobulin (β2m) gene, have greatly reduced numbers of CD4-CD8+ peripheral T cells.[118,119] In these knock-out mice lineage commitment of the double positive thymocytes has occurred independent of TCR-MHC class II or I interactions respectively. These observations support a stochastic/selective model for lineage commitment of immature double CD4CD8 positive thymocytes. In the stochastic/selective model, the CD4+CD8+ thymocyte randomly switches off either the CD4 or CD8 co-receptor, regardless of the specificity of its TCR. In the next set of differentiation steps, maturing thymocytes are positively selected via interactions of the TCR and co-receptor with MHC class I (CD8+) or class II (CD4+).[120]

Recently, evidence has been provided that maturing T cells which are not subjected to positive selection following engagement of the T-cell receptor and accessory molecules with MHC entities expressed in the thymic microenvironment, die through apoptosis.[121]

In conclusion, these studies involving the generation of the TCR repertoire show that the diversification process is not totally random but is controlled at several levels by selection processes during development and thymic selection. These various processes are not only influenced by the expressed MHC class I and II haplotypes but also

by other factors which are genetically predetermined and thus contribute to the shaping of the T-cell repertoire. In addition, both in
humans and mice there is ample evidence for thymocyte lineage commitment to occur on a stochastic basis. Subsequently, these maturing
single positive thymocytes are subjected to positive selection via TCR-
MHC class II or class I interactions.

1.5 ALLORECOGNITION

The mechanisms underlying T-cell recognition of allo-antigens are
not yet fully understood. The peripheral T-cell repertoire is shaped by
thymic selection processes and post-thymic modulations to be unre-
sponsive towards complexes of self MHC and self peptide but is responsive towards complexes of self MHC and foreign peptide or foreign MHC and peptide. The principle targets of the immune response
to allografts are the MHC molecules themselves, and T-cell recognition of allo-MHC is the primary and central event that initiates allograft rejection. There are currently two hypothesis which would explain the mechanism of T-cell recognition of allo-antigens (Fig. 1.5).
In the direct pathway of allorecognition the allogenic-MHC molecules
play a central role. T cells of the recipient are capable of recognizing
allo-MHC molecules themselves independent of peptide-binding or
peptide specificity[122-124] or complexes of allo-MHC and peptide.[125] These
peptides could be derived from endogenous proteins or from the MHC
molecules themselves.[20]

In the indirect pathway, T cells recognize processed allo-antigens
including allo-MHC molecules in the context of self-APC.[126-130] In this
way, a T-cell response is elicited that is restricted to the recipient's
own MHC molecules. Indirect recognition is expected to occur for
these allopeptides when presented by the recipient's MHC class II
molecules. The question remains as to whether and how the T-cell
repertoire involved in the direct pathway differs from that involved in
the indirect pathway (as will be discussed in chapter 3). Peptide elution studies for MHC class I and class II associated peptides have revealed the existence of MHC encoded peptides in the eluted pool.[20]
This shows that MHC derived peptides are processed and presented
by the MHC under normal circumstances. In humans, free HLA molecules have been found in the periphery of normal individuals. This
observation together with the observation of the existence of differently spliced MHC class I transcripts, which lack the transmembrane
region, suggests that in normal individuals these soluble HLA antigens
can be captured, endocytosed and processed by antigen presenting cells.
Consequently, MHC derived peptides can be presented by class II MHC
molecules and as a result play an important role in the shaping of the
$CD4^+CD8^-$ T-cell repertoire. In organ transplant patients soluble allo-
MHC antigens have been detected.[131,132] These allo-MHC antigens can
therefore be processed and presented as allopeptides by autologous MHC

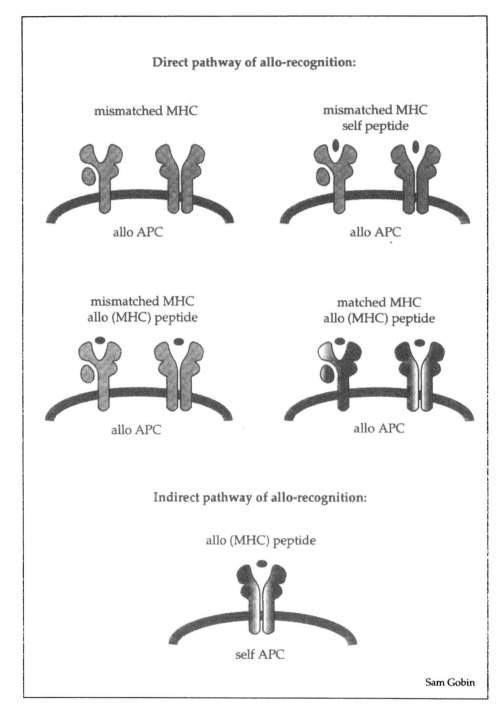

Fig. 1.5. Possible models for allorecognition. In the direct pathway the T-cell repertoire of the host is capable of recognizing mismatched allo-MHC molecules independent of peptide, dependent on allo-peptides or autologous peptides and matched allo-MHC and allo-peptides. In the indirect pathway autologous MHC class II molecules present allo (MHC) peptides.

class II molecules leading to T-cell recognition. Several studies have provided evidence now that T-cell recognition of processed allo-MHC peptides presented by self-MHC molecules does occur in vivo. T-cell recognition of MHC allopeptides presented by autologous MHC may therefore play a critical role in organ transplantation.[126,130,133-137]

The question remains whether the T-cell repertoire involved in the direct pathway differs from that involved in the indirect pathway. CTLp frequencies studies have revealed a relative high frequency of CTLp involved in the recognition of complexes of allo-MHC and peptide on the target cell. In these studies, individual specific differences in the CTLp frequency against similar MHC allo-antigens have been noted. Similarly, within individuals, the CTLp frequency against different allo-antigens varied.[138-140] This is probably the direct consequence of recognition of determinants on the allo-MHC and recognition of the entire pool of allopeptides. In contrast, recognition of allo-MHC derived peptides presented by autologous MHC is of less complexity which might be related to the restricted number of allo-MHC peptides that can be presented by autologous MHC.[133] In this regard, the frequency of self-restricted T cells is approximately 100-fold lower than that of T-cells recognizing intact allo-MHC.[141]

In conclusion, the direct pathway, where the T-cell receptor of allo-reactive T cells directly recognizes complete MHC molecules in the presence or absence of bound peptide, accounts for most of the cytotoxic T-cell function. In contrast, in the indirect pathway, where the T-cell receptor of alloreactive T cells recognizes MHC allopeptides after capture, processing and presentation by self-APCs, may account for much of the Th cell function. Consequently the T-cell receptor repertoires used in these various pathways may reveal different specificities.

1.6 Methodologies Currently Employed for the Analysis of TCR Repertoires

T-cell receptor analysis in transplantation

In transplantation, alloreactive T cells play an important role in the process of allograft rejection. Therefore, it seems feasible to assume that triggering of T cells by alloantigens expressed on the cell surface of the graft may lead to selective expansion of particular T cells which ultimately accumulate in the allograft. Various approaches are currently available to examine the nature of the T cell infiltrate in the allograft and of the circulating peripheral T-cell compartment in transplantation. These include T-cell receptor β-chain gene rearrangement studies on genomic DNA blots, analysis of T-cell receptor V gene expression at the transcriptional level by several PCR techniques and at the level of membrane expression of the T-cell receptor using monoclonal antibodies specific for TCR V-regions. Furthermore, the heterogeneity of the PCR amplified material can be assessed in a number of ways which include DNA sequence analysis; the application of single strand conformation polymorphism, spectratyping and immunoscope technologies.

1) TCR β chain rearrangement studies by the Southern blot technology

The first molecular TCR repertoire studies employed the Southern blot-technique to determine whether dominant TCR β-chain rearrangements could be detected in cell cultures of in vitro expanded tissue-infiltrating T lymphocytes.[142-144] In these studies TCR β-chain rearrangements were evaluated in Southern blots using DNA extracted from interleukin-2 (IL-2) propagated cells. This DNA was subjected to restriction endonuclease digestion usually with EcoRI and HindIII, permitting assessment of rearrangements to both TCRBC1 and TCRBC2. In such studies rearrangements shared among greater than 5% of the bulk culture appear as non germline bands, when hybridized with a TCRBC probe (see also chapter 4).

The outcome of these various studies yielded results ranging from clonal dominance to the presence of polyclonal T-cell populations on the basis of extensive TCR β-chain rearrangement patterns among biopsy derived T lymphocytes. It should be noted that these studies which showed dominant TCR β-chain rearrangement suggestive of clonal expansion of T lymphocytes in the allograft relied upon analysis of in vitro expansions of cell cultures in (IL-2) where selective clonal outgrowth could have influenced the outcome of the molecular analyses.[143-146] However, due to the sample size of the biopsy, Southern blot assessment of TCR β-chain rearrangements on freshly isolated material is hampered by the relative low numbers of graft-infiltrating T lymphocytes (GITL).

Alternatively, different T-cell clones may contain common TCRBD-TCRBJ rearrangements, which may result in a shared TCR β-chain rearrangement pattern.[147] Regarding this latter issue, several studies have now shown that gene elements of the TCRBJ2 locus, and in particular the TCRBJ2S1 and TCRBJ2S7 gene segments are preferentially incorporated in TCR β-chain rearrangements.[89-91,148-150] In either case, it cannot be excluded that the overall genomic size of TCR β-chain rearrangements might result from different TCRV-genes giving rise to similar sized restriction fragments. The question remains however whether the Southern blotting technique can properly discriminate between the differently rearranged fragments. In this respect, Kurnick et al., have recently studied a series of T-cell clones derived from synovial tissue of one rheumatoid artheritis (RA) patient.[151] These clones were selected because they shared a similar sized restriction fragment of a TCR β-chain rearrangement as suggested by the Southern blots. However, when an analysis of TCRV-gene usage was performed, it became clear that the clones were unrelated as they used different TCRV-genes.

2) Semi-quantitative analysis of TCRV-gene usage by the PCR-technique

In more recent studies, the PCR-technique was employed to analyze the TCRV-gene usage in biopsies to be compared to peripheral blood of transplant patients. For these analyses several PCR based approaches are currently available.

1. Single sided PCR-amplification, such as inverse and anchor PCR analysis[152-154] allows for analysis of TCRV-gene usage via DNA sequencing or hybridization with family specific oligonucleotides. By using this technique, the detection of previously undefined TCRV-region sequences is possible. However, a large number of TCR sequences need to be studied to obtain a representative picture of the overall TCR repertoire.

2. Semi-quantitative PCR-amplification using family specific TCRV-gene primers amplifying the selected V-gene families[155-158] allows for direct detection of individual TCRV-gene families. The amplified PCR product can also be sequenced to characterize the NDNJ region of the TCR. A drawback of this approach is that novel TCRV-gene sequences escape detection.

3. PCR-amplification using degenerate 5' primers that are able to anneal to a wide range of TCRV-gene sequences. The individual TCRV-genes used in TCR rearrangements can subsequently be identified via hybridization with TCR V-gene family specific oligonucleotides as probes.[159,160] It is noteworthy that the use of this technique on clonal material, yielded good results. However, the amplification of T-cell lines with the degenerate primer was less effective in that not all TCRV-genes present were amplified with the same efficiency (Struyk and Hawes et al., unpublished).

3) Single strand conformation polymorphism (SSCP)

Non-denaturing gel electrophoresis as a method for the detection of junctional diversity in rearranged T-cell receptor sequences has been applied to define the extent of T-cell heterogeneity.[161] Detection of junctional diversity is based on mobility shifts of polymerase chain reaction amplified rearranged T-cell receptor sequences as a result of nucleotide sequence polymorphism. Using non-denaturing gel electrophoresis, separation of double stranded (homoduplexes) and single stranded DNA molecules is achieved revealing the level of T-cell receptor diversity in a cell mixture. Additional information on the T-cell receptor diversity in a cell population might be achieved by the application of heteroduplex formation (Offermans et al., unpublished). This approach is discussed in more detail in chapter 4.

4) Spectratyping and immunoscope-based analysis of T-cell receptor repertoires

These types of analyses show the size distribution of CDR3 in TCR α and β chains. It is based on the PCR amplification of a relative short stretch of the recombined TCR α and β chains and the electrophoretic mobility of the amplified PCR products in denaturing polyacrylamide gels.[162,163] This approach reveals the complexity of the TCR α and β chain rearrangements in a mixture of T lymphocytes.

5) Monoclonal Antibodies

Repertoires of T-cell receptors expressed at the cell surface of T lymphocytes can be analyzed at the protein level by the application of monoclonal antibodies (MoAbs). These studies allow in principle for accurate estimation of the numbers of T-cell receptors expressed at the cell surface. These studies have been hampered in the past by the paucity of the number of available monoclonal antibodies specific for the various TCRV-gene families. More recently the number of TCRBV-family specific MoAbs has increased, allowing the identification at the protein level of the majority of the currently known TCRBV gene families whereas still only a few TCRAV family specific MoAbs are available. Although ultimately, analysis of TCR expression on the cell membrane by flow cytometry is what is important in relation to MHC/peptide complex recognition, these analyses are hampered by several criteria. First of all, although the number of TCRV-gene specific immune reagents is increasing, they are in general not directed against a common epitope within a given family. Consequently, these reagents, as they are currently available do not recognize all members within a given TCRV-gene family. Secondly, these types of analyses only provide information to the extent of usage of TCRV-genes. They are not informative for the analysis of the composition of the antigen binding site. Consequently, the nature of the expansion of the T lymphocyte infiltrate as to the level of clonality within the tissue-infiltrating population of T lymphocytes cannot be determined.

REFERENCES

1. Klein J. Natural History of the major histocompatibility complex. In: J. Wiley and Sons (eds). New York, 1989.
2. Geraghty DE. Structure of the HLA class I region and expression of its resident genes. Curr Opin Immunol 1993; 5:3-7.
3. Wei X and Orr HT. Differential expression of HLA-E, HLA-F and HLA-G transcripts in human tissue. Hum Immunol 1990; 29:131-42.
4. Bodmer JG, Marsh SG, Albert ED et al. Nomenclature for factors of the HLA system. Tissue Antigens 1994; 43:1-18.
5. Bjorkman PJ, Saper MA, Samraoui B et al. Structure of the human class I histocompatibility antigen, HLA-A2. Nature 1987; 329:506-12.

6. Saper MA, Bjorkman PJ, Wiley DC. Refined structure of the human histocompatibility antigen HLA-A2 at 2.6Å resolution. J Mol Biol 1991; 219:277-319.

7. Garrett TPJ, Saper MA, Bjorkman PJ et al. Specificity pockets for the side chains of peptide antigens in HLA-Aw68. Nature 1989; 342:692-96.

8. Madden DR, Gorga JC, Strominger JL et al. The three-dimensional structure of HLA-B27 at 2.1Å resolution suggests a general mechanism for tight peptide binding to MHC. Cell 1992; 70:1035-48.

9. Madden DR, Corga JC, Strominger JL et al. The structure of HLA-B27 reveals nonamer self-peptides bound in an extended conformation. Nature 1991; 35:321-25.

10. Guo H-C, Jardetzky TS, Garrett TPJ et al. Different length peptides bind to HLA-Aw68 similarly at their ends but bulge out in the middle. Nature 1992; 360:364-67.

11. Buxton SA, Benjamin RJ, Clayberger C et al. Anchoring pockets in human histocompatibility complex leukocyte antigen (HLA) class I molecules: analysis of the conserved B ("45") pocket of HLA-B27. J Exp Med 1992; 175:809-20.

12. Brown JH, Jardetzky TS, Gorga JC et al. Three-dimensional structure of the human class II histocompatibility antigen HLA-DR1. Nature 1993; 364:33-39.

13. Stern LJ, Brown JH, Jardetzky TS et al. Crystal structure of the human class II MHC protein HLA-DR1 complexed with an influenza virus peptide. Nature 1994; 368:215-21.

14. Engelhard VH. Structure of peptides associated with MHC class I molecules. Curr opinion in Immunol 1994; 6:13-23.

15. Huckzo EL Bodnar WM, Benjamin D et al. Characteristics of endogenous peptides eluted from the class I MHC molecule HLA-B7 determined by mass spectrometry and computer modeling. J Immunol 1993; 151:2572-87.

16. Engelhard VH, Appella E, Benjamin DC et al. Mass spectrometric analysis of peptides associated with the human class I MHC molecules HLA-A2.1 and HLA-B7 and Identification of structural features that determine binding. Chem Immunol 1993; 57:39-62.

17. Hunt DF, Henderson RA, Shabanowitz J et al. Characterization of Peptides Bound to the class I MHC molecule HLA-A2.1 by mass spectrometry. Science 1992; 255:1261-63.

18. DiBrino M, Parker KC, Shiloach J et al. Endogenous peptides bound to HLA-A3 possess a specific combination of anchor residues that permit identification of potential antigenic peptides. Proc Natl Acad Sci USA 1993; 90:1508-12.

19. Jardetzky TS, Lane WS, Robinson RA et al. Identification of self peptides bound to purified HLA-B27. Nature 1991; 353:326-29.

20. Rammensee HG, Friede T and Stevanovi S. MHC ligands and peptide motifs: first listing. Immunogenetics 1995; 41:178-28.

21. Den Haan JMM, Sherman NE, Blokland E et al. Identification of a guH disease-associated human minor histocompatibility antigen. Science 1995; in press.

22. Ruppert J, Grey HM, Sette A et al. Prominent role of secondary anchor residues in peptide binding to A2.1 molecules. Cell 1993; 74:929-37.

23. Falk K, Rötzschke O, Grahovac B et al. Peptide motifs of HLA-B35 and B37 molecules. Immunogenetics 1993; 38:161-62.

24. Falk K, Rötzschke O, Stevanovi S et al. Allele-specific motifs revealed by sequencing of self-peptides eluted from MHC molecules. Nature 1991; 351:290-96.

25. Hill AVS, Elvin J, Willis AC et al. Molecular analysis of the association of HLA-B53 and resistance to severe malaria. Nature 1992; 360:434-39.

26. Rötzschke O, Falk K, Stevanovic S et al. Peptide motifs of closely related HLA class I molecules encompass substantial differences. Eur J Immunol 1992; 22:2453-56.

27. Sutton J, Rowland-Jones S, Rosenberg W et al. A sequence pattern for peptides presented to cytotoxic T lymphocytes by HLA-B8 revealed by the analysis of epitopes and eluted peptides. Eur J Immunol 1993; 23:447-53.

28. Matsui M, Hioe CE and Frelinger JA. Roles of the six peptide binding pockets of the HLA-A2 molecule in allorecognition by human cytotoxic T-cell clones. Proc Natl Acad Sci USA 1993; 90:674-78.

29. Matsui M, Moots RJ, McMichael AJ et al. Significance of the six peptide-binding pockets of HLA-A2.1 in influenza A matrix peptide-specific cytotoxic T-lymphocyte reactivity. Hum Immunol 1994; 41:160-66.

30. Rötzschke O and Falk K. Origin, structure and motifs of naturally processed MHC class II ligands. Current opinion in Immunol. 1994; 6:45-51.

31. Henderson RA, Michel H, Sakaguchi K et al. HLA-A2.1 associated peptides from a mutant cell line: a second pathway of antigen presentation. Science 1992; 255:1264-66.

32. Wei ML and Cresswell P. HLA-A2 molecules in an antigen-processing mutant contain signal sequence-derived peptides. Nature 1992; 356:443-46.

33. Wölfel T, Van Pel A, Brichard V et al. Two tyrosinase nonapeptides recognized on HLA-A2 melanomas by autologous cytolytic T lymphocytes. Eur J Immunol 1994; 24:759-64.

34. Chicz RM, Urban RG, Gorga JC et al. Specificity and promiscuity among naturally processed peptides bound to HLA-DR alleles. J Exp Med 1993; 178:27-47.

35. Chicz RM, Urban RG, Lane WS et al. Predominant naturally processed peptides bound to HLA-DR1 are derived from MHC-related molecules and are heterogeneous in size. Nature 1992; 358:764-68.

36. Riberdy JM, Newcomb JR, Surman MJ et al. HLA-DR molecules from an antigen-processing mutant cell line are associated with invariant chain peptides. Nature 1992; 360:474-77.

37. Sette A, Ceman S, Kubo RT et al. Invariant Chain peptides in most HLA-DR molecules of an antigen-processing mutant. Science 1992; 258:1801-04.
38. Geluk A, Van Meijgaarden KE, Janson AMA et al. Functional analysis of DR17(DR3)-restricted mycobacterial T-cell epitopes reveals DR17-binding motif and enables the design of allele-specific competitor peptides. J Immunol 1992; 149:2864-71.
39. Hammer J, Takacs B and Sinigaglia F. Identification of a motif for HLA DR1 binding peptides using M13 display libraries. J Exp Med 1992; 176:1007-13.
40. Hammer J. Valsasnini P, Tolba K et al. Promiscuous and allele-specific anchors in HLA-DR-binding peptides. Cell 1993; 74:197-203.
41. Falk K, Rötzschke O, Stevanovi S et al. Pool sequencing of natural HLA-DR, DQ and DP ligands reveals detailed peptide motifs, constraints of processing and general rules. Immunogenetics 1994; 39:230-42.
42. Malcharek G, Falk K, Rötzschke O et al. Natural peptide ligand motifs of two HLA molecules associated with myasthenia gravis. Int Immunol 1993; 5:1229-37.
43. O'Sullivan D, Sidney J, Del Guerico M-F et al. Truncation analysis of several DR binding epitopes. J Immunol 1990; 146:1240-46.
44. O'Sullivan D, Arrhenius T, Sidney J et al. On the interaction of promiscuous antigenic peptides with different DR alleles. Identification of common structural motifs. J Immunol 1991; 147:2663-69.
45. Panina-Bordignon P, Tan A, Termijtelen A et al. Universally immunogenic T-cell epitopes: promiscuous binding to human MHC class II and promiscuous recognition by T cells. Eur J Immunol 1989; 19:2237-42.
46. Ho PC, Mutch DA, Winkel KD et al. Identification of two promiscuous T-cell epitopes from tetanus toxin. Eur J Immunol 1990; 20:477-83.
47. Momburg F, Ortiz-Navarrete V, Neefjes JJ et al. The proteasome subunits encoded by the major histocompatibility complex are not essential for antigen presentation. Nature 1991; 353: 664-67.
48. Arnold D, Driscoll J, Androlewicz M et al. Proteasome subunits encoded in the MHC are not generally required for the processing of peptides bound by MHC class I molecules. Nature 1992; 360:171-77.
49. Spies T, Cerundolo V, Colonna M et al. Presentation of viral antigen by MHC class I molecules is dependent on a putative peptide transporter heterodimer. Nature 1992; 355:644-46.
50. Powis SJ, Townsend ARM, Deverson EV et al. Restoration of antigen presentation to the mutant cell line RMA-S by an MHC-linked transporter. Nature 1991; 354:528-31.
51. Kelly A, Powis SH, Kerr L-A et al. Assembly and function of the two ABC transporter proteins encoded in the human major histocompatibility complex. Nature 1992; 355:641-44.
52. Kleymeer MJ, Kelly A, Geuze HJ et al. Location of MHC-encoded transporters in the endoplasmic reticulum and cis-Golgi. Nature 1992; 357:342-44.

53. Degen E and Williams DB. Participation of a novel 88-kD protein in the biogenesis of murine class I histocompatibility molecules. J Cell Biol 1991; 112:1099-1115.

54. Degen E, Cohen-Doyle MF and Williams DB. Dissociation of the p88 chaperone from major histocompatibility complex class I molecules requires both β2-microglobulin and peptide. J Exp Med 1992; 175:1653-61.

55. Anderson KS and Cresswell P. A role for calnexin (IP90) in the assembly of class II MHC molecules. EMBO J 1994; 13:675-82.

56. Schreiber KL, Bell MP, Huntoon CJ et al. Class II histocompatibility molecules associate with calnexin during assembly in the endoplasmic reticulum. Int Immunol 1994; 6:101-11.

57. Roche PA and Cresswell P. Invariant chain association with HLA-DR molecules inhibits immunogenic peptide binding. Nature 1990; 345:615-18.

58. Teyton L, O'Sullivan D, Dickson PW et al. Invariant chain distinguishes between the exogenous and endogenous antigen presentation pathways. Nature 1990; 348:39-44.

59. Newcomb JR and Cresswell P. Characterization of endogenous peptides bound to parified HLA-DR molecules and their absence from invariant chain associated αβ dimers. J Immunol 1993; 150:499-507.

60. Anderson MS and Miller J. Invariant chain can function as a chaperone protein for class II major histocompatibility complex molecules. Proc Natl Acad Sci USA 1992; 89:2282-86.

61. Layet C and Germain RN. Invariant chain promotes egress of poorly expressed, haplotype mismatched class II major histocompatibility complex AaAβ dimers from the endoplasmic reticulum/cis-Golgi compartment. Proc Natl Acad Sci USA 1991; 88:2346-50.

62. Neefjes JJ, Stollorz V, Peters PJ et al. The biosynthetic pathway of MHC class II but not class I molecules intersects the endocytic route. Cell 1990; 61:171-183.

63. Bakke O and Dobberstein B. MHC class II-associated invariant chain contains a sorting signal for endosomal compartments. Cell 1990; 63:707-16.

64. Lotteau V, Teyton L, Peleraux A et al. Intracellular transport of class II MHC molecules directed by invariant chain. Nature 1990; 348:600-05.

65. Lamb CA, Yewdell JW, Bennink JR et al. Invariant chain targets HLA class II molecules to acidic endosomes containing internalized influenza virus. Proc Natl Acad Sci USA 1991; 88:5889-6002.

66. Pieters J, Horstmann H, Bakke O et al. Intracellular transport and localization of major histocompatibility complex class II molecules and associated invariant chain. J Cell Biol 1991; 115:1213-23.

67. Peters PJ, Neefjes JJ, Oorschot V et al. Segregation of MHC class II molecules from MHC class I molecules in the Golgi complex for transport to lysosomal compartments. Nature 1991; 349:669-76.

68. Harding CV, Collins DS, Slot JW et al. Liposome-encapsulated antigens are processed in lysosomes, recycled and presented to T cells. Cell 1991; 64:393-401.

69. Neefjes JJ and Ploegh HL. Inhibition of endosomal proteolytic activity by leupeptin blocks surface expression of MHC class II molecules and their conversion to SDS resistant αβ heterodimers in endosomes. EMBO J 1992; 11:411-16.

70. Blum JS and Cresswell P. Role for intracellular proteases in the processing and transport of class II HLA antigens. Proc Natl Acad Sci USA 1988; 85:3975-79.

71. Davis MM and Bjorkman PJ. T-cell antigen receptor genes and T-cell recognition. Nature 1988; 334:395-402.

72. Chothia C, Boswell DR and Lesk AM. The outline structure of the T cell αβreceptor. EMBO J 1988; 7:3745-55.

73. Claverie J-M, Prochnicka-Chalufour A and Bougueleret L. Implications of a Fab-like structure for the T-cell receptor. Immunol Today 1989; 10:10-14.

74. Benoist C and Mathis D. Positive selection of the T cell repertoire: where and when does it occur? Cell 1989; 58:1027-33.

75. Bill J and Palmer E. Positive selection of CD4+ T cells mediated by MHC class II bearing stromal cell in thymic cortex. Nature 1989; 341:649-51.

76. Gulwani-Akolkar B, Posnett DM, Janson CH et al. T-cell receptor V segment frequencies in peripheral blood T cells correlate with human leukocyte antigen type. J Exp Med 1991; 174:1139-46.

77. Reed EF, Tugulea SL and Suciu-Forca N. Influence of HLA class I and class II antigens on the peripheral T-cell repertoire. Hum Immunol 1994; 40:111-22.

78. Genevée C, Farace F, Chung V et al. Influence of human leukocyte antigen genes on TCR V gene segment frequencies. Int Immunol 1994; 6:1497-04.

79. Akolkar PN, Gulwani-Alkokar B, Pergolizzi R et al. Influence of HLA genes on T-cell receptor V segment frequencies and expression levels in peripheral blood lymphocytes. J Immunol 1993; 150:2761-73.

80. Loveridge JA, Rosenburg WMC, Kirkwood TBL et al. The genetic contribution to human T-cell receptor repertoire. Immunol 1991; 74:246-50.

81. Moss PAH, Rosenberg WMC, Zintzaras E et al. Characterization of the human T-cell receptor α-chain repertoire and demonstration of a genetic influence on Vα usage. Eur J Immunol 1993; 23: 1153-59.

82. Hawes GE, Struyk L and Van den Elsen PJ. Differential usage of T-cell receptor V gene segments in CD4+ and CD8+ subsets of T lymphocytes in monozygotic twins. J Immunol 1993; 150:2033-45.

83. Grunewald J, Janson CH and Wigzell H. Biased expression of individual T-cell receptor V gene segments in CD4+ and CD8+ human peripheral blood T lymphocytes. Eur J Immunol 1991; 21:819-22.

84. Gulwani-Akolkar B, Posnett D.N, Janson C.H et al. T-cell receptor V segment frequencies in peripheral blood T cells correlate with human leukocyte antigen type. J Exp Med 1991; 174: 1139-46.

85. Liao N-S, Maltzman J and Raulet D. Expression of the Vβ5.1 gene by murine peripheral T cells is controlled by MHC genes and skewed to the CD8+ subset. J Immunol 1990; 144: 844-48.

86. Davey MP, Meyer MM, Munkirs M et al. T-cell receptor variable β genes show differential expression in CD4+ and CD8+ cells. Hum Immunol 1991; 32:194-207.

87. Singer PA, Balderas RS and Theofilopoulos AN. Thymic selection defines multiple T cell receptor Vβ "repertoire phenotypes" at the CD4/CD8 subset level. EMBO J 1990; 9:3641-36.

88. Candeias S, Waltzinger C, Benoist C et al. The Vβ17+ T-cell repertoire: skewed Jβ usage after thymic selection; dissimilar CDR3s in CD4+ versus CD8+ cells. J Exp Med 1991; 174: 989-1000.

89. Jeddi-Tehrani M, Grunewald J, Hodara V et al. Nonrandom T-cell receptor Jβ usage pattern in human CD4+ and CD8+ peripheral T cells. Hum Immunol 1994; 40: 93-100.

90. Grunewald J, Jeddi-Tehrani M, Pisa E et al. Analysis of Jβ gene segment usage by CD4+ and CD8+ human peripheral blood T lymphocytes. Int Immunol 1992; 4: 643-50.

91. Raaphorst FM, Kaijzel EL, Van Tol MJD et al. Non-random employment of Vβ6 and Jβ gene elements and conserved amino acid usage profiles in CDR3 regions of human fetal and adult TCR β chain rearrangements. Int Immunol. 1994; 6:1-9.

92. Robinson MA. Usage of human T-cell receptor Vβ, Jβ, Cβ and Vα gene segments is not proportional to gene number. Hum Immunol 1992; 35:60-67.

93. George JF and Schroeder HW. Developmental regulation of Dβ reading frame and junctional diversity in T-cell receptor-β transcripts from human thymus. J Immunol 1992; 148: 1230-39.

94. Feeney AJ. Junctional sequences of fetal T cell receptor β chains have few N regions. J Exp Med 1991; 174:115-24.

95. Prochnicka-Chalufour A, Casanova JL, Avrameas S et al. Biased amino acid distributions in regions of the T cell receptors and MHC molecules potentially involved in their association. Int Immunol 1991; 3:853-64.

96. Fink PJ and Bevan MJ. H2 antigens of the thymus determine lymphocyte specificity. J Exp Med 1978; 148:766-75.

97. Zinkernagel RM, Callahan GN, Althaga A et al. On the thymus in differentiation of "H-2 self recognition" by T cells: evidence for dual recognition? J Exp Med 1978; 147:882-96.

98. Sprent J, Lo D, Gao EK et al. T-cell selection in the thymus. Immunol Rev 1988; 101:173-90.

99. Schwartz RH. Acquisition of immunologic self-tolerance. Cell 1989; 57:1073-81.

100. Nikolic-Zugic J and Bevan MJ. Role of self-peptides in positively selecting the T-cell repertoire. Nature 1990; 344:65-67.

101. Mombaerts P, Clarke AR, Rudnicki MA et al. Mutations in T-cell antigen receptor genes α and β block thymocyte development at different stages. Nature 1992; 360:225-31.

102. Kishi H, Borgulya P, Scott B et al. Surface expression of the β T-cell receptor (TCR) chain in the absence of other TCR or CD3 proteins on immature T cells. EMBO J 1991; 10:93-100.

103. Goettrup M, Baron A, Griffiths G et al. T-cell receptor (TCR) β chain homodimers on the surface of immature but not mature α, γ, δ chain deficient T-cell lines. EMBO J 1992; 11:2735-46.

104. Groettrup M, Ungewiss K, Azogui O et al. A novel disulfide-linked heterodimer on pre-T cells consists of the T-cell receptor β chain and a 33 kd glycoprotein. Cell 1993; 75:283-94.

105. Kisielow P, Teh HS, Bluthmann H et al. Positive selection of antigen-specific T cells in thymus by restricting MHC molecules. Nature 1988; 335:730-33.

106. Sha WC, Nelson CA, Newberry RD et al. Positive and negative selection of an antigen receptor on T cells in transgenic mice. Nature 1988; 336:73-76.

107. Borgulya P, Kisyi H, Müller U et al. Development of the CD4 and CD8 lineage of T cells: instruction versus selection. EMBO J 1991; 10:913-18.

108. Kaye J, Hsu ML, Sauron ME et al. Selective development of CD4⁺ T cells in transgenic mice expressing a class II MHC-restricted antigen receptor. Nature 1989; 341:746-49.

109. Marrack P, Lo D, Brinster R et al. The effect of thymus environment on T-cell development and tolerance. Cell 1988; 53:627-34.

110. Von Boehmer H. Thymic selection: a matter of life and death. Immunol Today 1992; 12:454-58.

111. Robey E, Ramsdell F, Elliott J et al. Expression of CD4 in transgenic mice alters the specificity of CD8 cells for allogenic major histocompatibility complex. Proc Natl Acad Sci USA 1991; 88:608-12.

112. Teh HS, Garvin AM, Forbush KA et al. Participation of CD4 coreceptor molecules in T-cell repertoire selection. Nature 1991; 349: 241-43.

113. Kruisbeek AM, Mond JJ, Fowlkes BJ et al. Absence of the lyt-2-,L3T4⁺ lineage of T cells in mice treated neonatally with anti-I-A correlates with absence of intrathymic I-A-bearing antigen-presenting cell function. J Exp Med 1985; 161:1029-47.

114. Kruisbeek AM, Fultz MK, Sharrow SO et al. Early development of the T-cell repertoire. In vivo treatment of neonatal mice with anti-Ia antibodies interferes with differentiation of I-restricted T cells but not K/D-restricted T cells. J Exp Med 1983; 157:1932-46.

115. Zuñiga-Pflucker JC, Longo DL and Kruisbeek AM. Positive selection of CD4⁻ CD8⁺ T cell in the thymus of normal mice. Nature 1989; 338:76-78.

116. Cosgrove D, Gray D, Dierich A et al. Mice lacking MHC class II molecules. Cell 1991; 66:1051-66.

117. Grusby MJ, Johnson RS, Papaioannou VE et al. Depletion of CD4⁺ T cells in major histocompatibility complex class II-deficient mice. Science 1991; 253: 1417-20.

118. Zijlstra M, Bix M, Simister NE et al. β2-Microglobulin deficient mice lack CD4⁻8⁺ cytolytic T cells. Nature 1990; 344:742-46.

119. Koller BH, Marrack P, Kappler JW et al. Normal development of mice deficient in β2-m, MHC class I proteins and CD8⁺ T cells. Science 1990; 248:1227-30.

120. Chan SH, Cosgrove D, Waltzinger C et al. Another view of the selective model of thymocyte selection. Cell 1993; 73:225-36.
121. Surh C and Sprent J. T-cell apoptosis detected in situ during positive and negative selection in the thymus. Nature 1994; 372:100-03.
122. Elliot TJ and Eisen HN. Cytotoxic T lymphocytes recognize a reconstituted class I histocompatibility antigen (HLA-A2) as an allogenic target molecule. Proc Natl Acad Sci USA 1990; 87:5213-17.
123. Bevan MJ. High determinant density may explain the phenomenon of alloreactivity. Immunol. Today 1984; 5:128-30.
124. Müllbacher A, Hill AB, Blanden RV et al. Alloreactive cytotoxic T cells recognize MHC class I antigen without peptide specificity. J Immunol 1991; 147:1765-72.
125. Lechler RI, Lombardi G, Batchelor JR et al. The molecular basis of alloreactivity. Immunol. Today 1990; 11:83-88.
126. Benichou G, Takizawa PA, Olson CA et al. Donor major histocompatibility complex (MHC) peptides are presented by recipients MHC molecules during graft rejection. J Exp Med 1992; 175:305-08.
127. Parker KE, Dalchau R, Fowler VJ et al. Stimulation of CD4+ T lymphocytes by allogeneic MHC peptides presented an autologous antigen-presenting cells. Transplantation 1992; 53:918-24.
128. Chen BP, Madrigal JA and Parham P. Cytotoxic T-cell recognition of an endogenous class I HLA peptide by a class II HLA molecule. J Exp Med 1990; 172:779-88.
129. Sherwood RA, Brent L and Rayfield LS. Presentation of alloantigens by host cells. Eur J Immunol 1986; 16:569-74.
130. Liu Z, Braunstein NS and Suciu-Foca N. T-cell recognition of allopeptides in context of syngeneic MHC. J Immunol 1992; 148:35-40.
131. Davies HS, Pollard SG and Calne RY. Soluble HLA antigens in the circulation of liver graft recipients. Transplantation 1989; 47:524-27.
132. Zavazava N, Böttcher H, Müller Ruchholtz W. Soluble MHC class I antigens (sHLA) and anti-HLA antibodies in heart and kidney allograft recipients. Tissue Antigens 1993; 42:20-26.
133. Benichou G, Fedoseyeva E, Lehmann PV et al. Limited T-cell response to donor MHC peptides during allograft rejection. J Immunol 1994; 153:938-45.
134. Fangmann J, Dalchau R and Fabre JW. Rejection of skin allografts by indirect allorecognition of donor class I major histocompatibility complex peptides. J Exp Med 1992; 175:1521-29.
135. Fangmann J, Dalchau R, Sawyer GJ et al. T-cell recognition of donor major histocompatibility complex class I peptides during allograft rejection. Eur J Immunol 1992; 22:1525-30.
136. Sayegh MH, Khoury SK, Hancock WW et al. Induction of immunity and oral tolerance with polymorphic class II MHC allopeptides. Proc Natl Acad Sci USA 1992; 89:7762-66.
137. De Koster HS, Anderson DE and Termijtelen A. T cells sensitized to synthetic HLA-DR3 peptide give evidence of continuous presentation of denatured HLA-DR3 molecules. J Exp Med 1989; 169:1191-96.

138. Sharrock C, Man S, Wanachiwanawin W et al. Analysis of the alloreactive T-cell repertoire in man. I. Differences in precursor frequency for cytotoxic T-cell responses against allogeneic MHC molecules in unrelated individuals. Transplantation 1987; 43:699-703.

139. Zhang L, Li S, Vandekerckhove BAE et al. Analysis of cytotoxic T-cell precursor frequencies directed against individual HLA-A and HLA-B alloantigens. J Immunol Meth 1989; 121: 39-45.

140. Man S, Lechler RI, Batchelor JR et al. Individual variation in the frequency of HLA class II-specific cytotoxic T-lymphocyte precursors. Eur J Immunol 1990; 20:847-54.

141. Liu Z, Sun Y, Xi Y et al. Contribution of direct and indirect recognition pathways to T-cell alloreactivity. J Exp Med 1993; 177:1643-50.

142. Stamenkovic I, Stegagno M, Wright KA et al. Clonal dominance among T lymphocyte infiltrates in arthritis. Proc Natl Acad Sci USA 1988; 85:1179-83.

143. Miceli MC and Finn OJ. T-cell receptor β-chain selection in human allograft rejection. J Immunol 1989; 142:81-86.

144. Frisman DM, Hurwitz AA, Bennett WT et al. Clonal analysis of graft-infiltrating lymphocytes from renal and cardiac biopsies. Dominant rearrangements of TCRβ genes and persistence of dominant rearrangements in serial biopsies. Hum Immunol 1990; 28:208-15.

145. Hand SL, Hall BL and Finn OJ. T-cell receptor gene usage and expression in enal allograft-derived T-cell lines. Hum Immunol 1990; 28:82-95.

146. Finn OJ and Miceli MC. Effector T-cell repertoire selection in human allograft rejection. Transplant Proc 1989; 21:346-48.

147. Duby AD, Sinclair AK, Osborne-Lawrence SL et al. Clonal heterogeneity of synovial fluid T lymphocytes from patients with rheumatoid arthritis. Proc Natl Acad Sci USA 1989; 86:6206-10.

148. Kronenberg M, Siu G, Hood L et al. The molecular genetics of the T-cell antigen receptor and T-cell antigen recognition. Ann Rev Immunol 1986; 4: 529-91.

149. Moss PAH, Rosenberg WMC and Bell JI. The human T-cell receptor in health and disease. Annu Rev Immunol 1992; 10:71-96.

150. Rosenberg WMC, Moss PAH and Bell JI. Variation in human T-cell receptor Vβ and Jβ repertoire: analysis using anchor polymerase chain reaction. Eur J Immunol 1992; 22: 541-49.

151. Struyk L, Hawes GE, Chatilla MK et al. T-cell receptors in rheumatoid arthritis. Arthr and Rheum 1995, 5:557-589.

152. Loh EY, Elliott JF, Cwirla S et al. Polymerase chain reaction with single-sided specificity: analysis of T-cell receptor δ chain. Science 1989; 243:217-20.

153. Ohara O, Dorit RL and Gilbert W. One-sided polymerase chain reaction: the amplification of cDNA. Proc Natl Acad Sci USA 1989; 86:5673-77.

154. Uematsu Y, Wege H, Straus A et al. The T-cell receptor repertoire in the synovial fluid of a patient with rheumatoid arthritis is polyclonal. Proc Natl Acad Sci USA 1991; 88:8534-38.

155. Struyk L, Kurnick JT, Hawes GE et al. T-cell receptor V gene usage in synovial fluid lymphocytes of patients with chronic arthritis. Hum Immunol 1993; 37: 237-51.

156. Oksenberg JR, Stuart S, Begovich AB et al. Limited heterogeneity of re-arranged T-cell receptor Vα transcripts in brains of multiple sclerosis patients. Nature 1990; 345:344-46.

157. Choi Y, Kotzin B, Herron L et al. Interaction of *Staphylococcus aureus* toxin "superantigens" with human T cells. Proc Natl Acad Sci USA 1989; 86:8941-8945.

158. Wucherpfennig KW, Ota K, Endo N et al. Shared human T-cell receptor Vβ usage to immunodominant regions of myelin basic protein. Science 1990; 248:1016-19.

159. Sottini A, Imberti L, Bettinardi A et al. Selection of T lymphocytes in two rheumatoid arthritis patients defines different T-cell receptor Vβ repertoires in CD4⁺ and CD8⁺ T-cell subsets. J Autoimmunity 1993; 6:621-37.

160. Broeren CPM, Verjans GMGM, Van Eden W et al. Conserved nucleotide sequences at the 5' end of T-cell receptor variable genes facilitate polymerase chain reaction amplification. Eur J Immunol 1991; 21:569-75.

161. Orita M, Suzuki Y, Sekiya T et al. Rapid and sensitive detection of point mutations and DNA polymorphisms using the polymerase chain reaction. Genomics 1989; 5:874-79.

162. Pannetier C, Cochet M, Darche S et al. The sizes of the CDR3 hypervariable regions of the muringe T-cell receptor β chains vary as a function of the recombined germ-line segments. Proc Natl Acad Sci USA 1993; 90:4319-23.

163. Gorski J, Yassai M, Zhu X et al. Circulating T-cell repertoire complexity in normal individuals and bone marrow recipients analyzed by CDR3 size spectratyping. Correlation with immune status. J Immunol 1994; 152:5109-19.

CHAPTER 2

THE CIRCULATING HUMAN PERIPHERAL T-CELL REPERTOIRE

Linda Struyk, Gail E. Hawes,
Frank Raaphorst, Marja van Eggermond,
Barbara Godthelp and Peter J. van den Elsen

2. ABSTRACT

The mechanisms controlling the generation of T-cell receptor repertoire and T-cell receptor selection are not clearly understood and seem to occur in an apparently random manner. To address the question to what extent the T-cell receptor repertoire is randomly shaped, i.e. antigen driven or is subject to individual specific genetic influences, we have carried out several studies. These studies included the analysis of the degree of combinatorial diversification in both the $CD4^+CD8^-$ and $CD4^-CD8^+$ subsets of T-lymphocytes in monozygotic twins and HLA non-identical, unrelated individuals. Furthermore, we have also analyzed the development of the T-cell receptor repertoire during fetal life and have evaluated the degree of junctional diversification in great detail within several TCRV-regions expressed by circulating peripheral blood T-lymphocytes by DNA sequence analysis of the CDR3 regions. These studies have led to the following conclusions:

1. The predominant influence shaping the T-cell receptor repertoire is genetically predetermined, of which HLA-predicted selection mechanisms exerted during thymic maturation are important contributing factors.
2. In the periphery, the available T-cell receptor repertoires are seemingly smaller than expected on the basis of non-random

The Human T-Cell Receptor Repertoire and Transplantation, edited by Peter J. van
den Elsen. © 1995 R.G. Landes Company.

usage of TCRBV and TCRBJ elements and amino acid composition of the CDR3 regions.
3. Within the CDR3 regions individual-specific amino acid motifs can be discerned.

2.1 INTRODUCTION

The T-cell receptor complex confers immunity by the specific recognition of foreign antigenic peptides in the context of self-MHC molecules.[1-4] The T-cell receptor complex is a multi protein ensemble which on the cell membrane consists in most cases of the clonotypic αβ T-cell receptor heterodimer in non-covalent association with the CD3 complex.[5,6] Both the α and β chain of the T-cell receptor consist of a variable and a constant domain. The antigen specificity of the T-cell receptor resides in the variable domain which is generated during thymic maturation by recombination through somatic rearrangement of germline encoded TCRV (variable), TCRD (diversity, β chain only) and TCRJ (joining) gene segments. The extent of the diversity of the T-cell receptor is determined by the number of possible combinations of TCRV, TCRD (β chain only) and TCRJ segments that can be employed in T-cell receptor rearrangements. Further diversification is achieved during recombination through additional mechanisms which operate on the TCRAV-TCRAJ and TCRBV-TCRBD-TCRBJ joinings. These include the random removal of coding nucleotides from the TCRV, (TCRD) and TCRJ elements and the addition of template independent nucleotides (N-nucleotides) or template-dependent P-nucleotides during V(D)J recombination.[7-9]

Based on the overall sequence homology with immunoglobin (Ig) molecules, the T-cell receptor has been proposed to fold into an Ig-like structure.[3,10-14] In the T-cell receptor, three regions of hypervariability can be discerned (the so-called complementarity determining regions, designated CDR1, CDR2 and CDR3), which together form the antigen binding site. the CDR1 and CDR2 regions are encoded by the T-cell receptor V-elements and are thought to interact with the α-helices in the MHC molecule. In analogy with the structure of Ig molecules, the V(D)J junction of the T-cell receptor encodes the CDR3 region which interacts with the peptide bound in the MHC molecule.[3,12-14]

Although the peripheral T-cell receptor repertoire is potentially extremely diverse, there is evidence which suggests that the actual peripheral T-cell receptor repertoire is in fact smaller than the potential T-cell receptor repertoire. This is related to the fact that the usage of TCRAV and TCRBV families in peripheral blood T lymphocytes has been shown to be subject to individual-specific and T-cell subset related differences.[15-21] Also the usage of the TCRBJ segments is not random; the TCRBJ2 gene segments, in general, are used at higher frequencies in TCR β chain rearrangements in comparison to TCRBJ1 gene segments.[18,22] Furthermore, in a number of studies skewing of individual TCRBJ segments in CD4⁺CD8⁻ or CD4⁻CD8⁺ T cells was noted.[23,24] Besides, it has been shown that certain TCR α and TCR β chains may not be able to form αβ TCR heterodimers.[25] In addition, mapping analysis of the 24 TCRBV families revealed that 10% of the TCRBV elements are not involved in productive rearrangements.[26]

To gain insight in the composition of a normal circulating peripheral T-cell receptor repertoire, we have analyzed the expression of TCRAV and TCRBV regions in peripheral blood T-lymphocytes of healthy donors to determine the extent of the diversity of the T-cell receptor repertoire both at the level of combinatorial and junctional diversity. Our studies have led to the conclusion that the actual peripheral T-cell receptor repertoire is seemingly smaller than expected on the basis of random usage of gene elements which make-up the TCR V-regions. Although the MHC by virtue of its ability to present peptides, plays an important role in the shaping of the peripheral T-cell receptor repertoire, there is evidence to suggest that the shaping of the peripheral T-cell receptor repertoire is also under the influence of individual specific, genetically predetermined factors.

2.2 RESULTS

EXPRESSION OF TCRAV AND TCRBV GENE FAMILIES IN PERIPHERAL BLOOD DERIVED T-LYMPHOCYTES

To analyze the TCRAV and TCRBV repertoires of T-lymphocytes among peripheral blood mononuclear cells (PBMC), T cells were recovered by Ficoll-Isopaque gradient centrifugation. RNA was extracted from freshly isolated PBMC of three HLA non-identical unrelated donors and was used for the determination of the TCRAV and TCRBV repertoires at the transcriptional level by a semiquantitative RT-PCR method both with TCRAV and TCRBV family specific oligonucleotides. The HLA type of the donors is depicted in Table 2.1. This approach allows us to determine the relative TCRAV and TCRBV gene usage frequencies among PBMC. The sequences of the TCRAV and TCRBV specific oligonucleotides used by our laboratory are shown in Table 2.2. An example of such a TCR V-gene RT-PCR analysis is presented in Figure 2.1. Almost all TCRAV and TCRBV gene segments tested for could be detected among PBMC of these individuals. The amounts of PCR product of each individual TCRAV and TCRBV gene family varied among the different individuals used in our analyses. In general the TCRAV2, V3, V8, V12 and V16 were the most frequently employed TCRAV-gene families. In a similar fashion the TCRBV2, V3, V4, V5, V6, V7, V8, V14 and V19 genes were in general dominant among PBMC derived T-lymphocytes. Of the various TCRBV gene families, the TCRBV10 and TCRBV11 were usually infrequently employed by peripheral blood derived T lymphocytes. The usual low intensity of the PCR product of the TCRBV10 and TCRBV11 gene families as detected after hybridization with a TCRBC probe was not the result of a less efficient amplification potential of the TCRBV10 and TCRBV11 oligonucleotides since our primers amplified TCRBV10 and TCRBV11 sequences from individual T-cell clones at a similar rate as the other TCRBV-gene family specific oligonucleotides used in our analyses. Taking into account the number of germ-line copies of TCRAV and TCRBV gene segments, quantitative variations in TCRAV and TCRBV gene usage as observed are likely the result of differences in the level of TCRAV and TCRBV gene transcription and assessibility of some of the TCRAV and TCRBV genes to the recombination process.

USAGE OF TCRAV AND TCRBV GENE FAMILIES IN HUMAN FETAL TCR REARRANGEMENTS

To gain insight into the generation of the αβ TCR repertoire and possible developmental influences on the usage of TCR V gene families during the establishment of the human TCR A and B repertoire we have investigated the usage of TCRAV and TCRBV gene families in TCR rearrangements derived from fetal peripheral tissues including cord blood, the primary hematopoietic organs and thymi. Figure 2.2 shows the results of the Southern blot analyses of the expression of TCRAV and TCRBV gene families in fetal cord blood (CB) at 13 weeks of gestation in comparison to PBMC of a healthy donor. As can be seen most of the TCRAV and TCRBV gene families were expressed at 13 weeks of gestation in fetal cord blood (Raaphorst et al.[27]). In a similar fashion, when fetal thymi (FT) at 17 weeks of gestation, and pediatric thymi (AT) were compared it was found that most of the TCRAV and TCRBV gene families were employed in TCR rearrangements

Table 2.1. HLA-type of donors

| Donors | Sex | HLA-type | |
		Class I	Class II
1	F	A3, A11, B7, B16, B39, (Bw6), Cw7	DR1, DR7, DR3 DQ1, DQ2
2	F	A2, A11, B15, B62, B35, (Bw6) Cw3, Cw4	DR1, DR4, DR53, DQ1, DQ3, DQ7
3	F	A2, B12, B44, (Bw4) B15, B62, (Bw6) Cw4	DR2, DR15, DR4, DR53 DQ1, DQ6, DQ3, DQ8

The HLA type of the individuals was determined by standard serological HLA-typing.

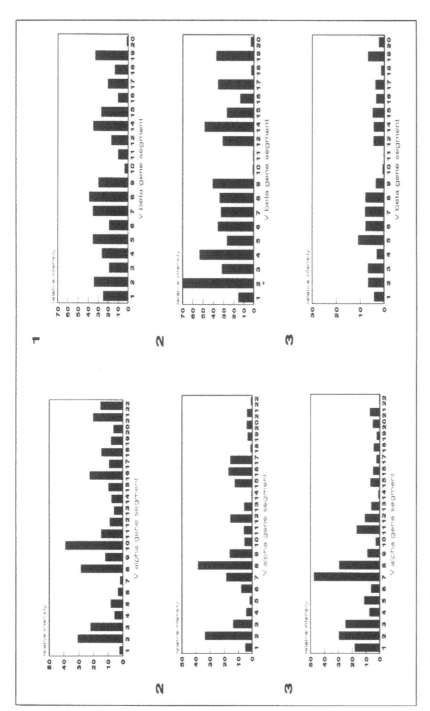

Fig. 2.1. TCRAV and TCRBV repertoire in PBMC. PBMC were obtained by Ficoll/Isopaque density gradient centrifugation. RNA was extracted with RNAzol (Cinna/Biotecx Laboratories, Houston, TX, U.S.A.). Five µg of total RNA was used for random or oligo dT-primed cDNA synthesis system (Promega Corp., Madison, WI, USA). The cDNA was diluted to 100 µl H₂O and 1 µl per reaction was used in PCR-amplifications with 20 pmol each of the TCRAV and TCRBV family specific 5' sense primers and a 3' antisense TCRAC or TCRBC primer accordingly (see Table 2.2). As internal control for total amplification and for normalization of the PCR-products, a reaction tube containing an internal 5' sense and the 3' antisense C region primers was included. The PCR was performed as previously described by Hawes et al.[20] and Struyk et al.[67] An aliquot of the amplified products of the TCRV gene segments and serial dilutions of the C gene segment were size separated in a 1% agarose gel and transferred to nylon membranes (Biotrace RP or HP, Gelman Sciences, Ann Arbor, MI. U.S.A.). The membranes were hybridized with ³²P radio labeled TCR Cα or Cβ specific probes and the autoradiograms were analyzed by densitometry (LKB 2220-020, Ultrascan XL, Laser Densitometer) to measure the intensity of the bands to achieve a relative value for the amount of amplification.

Table 2.2. TCR family-specific oligonucleotides for the TCR α and β chain

	5'　　　　　　　　　　　　　3'	CLONE
TCRAV1	TTG.CCC.TGA.GAG.ATG.CCA.GAG	HAP10
TCRAV2	GTG.TTC.CAG.AGG.GAG.CCA.TTG.CC	HAP26
TCRAV3	GGT.GAA.CAG.TCA.ACA.GGG.AGA	HAP05
TCRAV4	AAG.ACA.GAA.AGT.CCA.GTA.CCT.TGA.TCC.TGC	HAP08
TCRAV5	GGC.CCT.GAA.CAT.TCA.GGA	HAP35
TCRAV6	GTC.ACT.TTC.TAG.CCT.GCT.GA	HAP01
TCRAV7	AGG.AGC.CAT.TGT.CCA.GAT.AAA	HAP21
TCRAV8	GGA.GAG.AAT.GTG.GAG.CAG.CAT.C	HAP41
TCRAV9	ATC.TCA.GTG.CTT.GTG.ATA.ATA	HAP36
TCRAV10	AAT.TCT.CCG.TGT.CCA.TTC.TTT.GGA	HAP58
TCRAV11	AGA.AAG.CAA.GGA.CCA.AGT.GTT	HAP02
TCRAV12	CAG.AAG.GTA.ACT.CAA.GCG.CAG.ACT	PGA5
TCRAV13	TGC.TGT.GTG.AGA.GGA.ATA.CAA.GTG	HAVT15
TCRAV14	GAT.CTC.CAC.CTG.TCT.TGA.ATT.TAG	HAVT20
TCRAV15	CAG.AGT.CTT.TTC.CTG.AGT.GTC.CGA.G	HAVT31
TCRAV16	GAG.TGG.GCT.GAG.AGC.TCA.GTC.AGT.G	HAVT32
TCRAV17	GCT.TAT.GAG.AAC.ACT.GCG.T	AB11
TCRAV18	GCA.GCT.TCC.CTT.CCA.GCA.AT	AB21
TCRAV19	AGA.ACC.TGA.CTG.CCC.AGG.AA	AC24
TCRAV20	CAT.CTC.CAT.GGA.CTC.ATA.TGA	AF212
TCRAV21	GAC.TAT.ACT.AAC.AGC.ATG.T	AF211
TCRAV22	ATG.TCA.GGC.AAT.GAC.AAG.GGA.AGC	AC9
TCRAV23	CAG.GAG.GTG.ACA.CAG.ATT.CC	IGRa01
TCRAV24	GAT.CAT.CCT.GGA.GGG.AAA.GA	IGRa02
TCRAV25	GGT.CAA.CAG.CTG.AAT.CAG.CC	IGRa03
TCRAV26	TCA.GTC.CTT.GAT.CGT.CCA.AG	IGRa04
TCRAV27	TCT.GTT.CCT.GAG.CAT.GCA.GG	IGRa05
TCRAV28	TCT.ATC.TCT.GGT.TGT.CCA.CG	IGRa06
TCRAV29	TCA.AGC.CGT.GAT.CCT.CCG.AG	IGRa07
5'TCRAC	GAA.CCC.TGA.CCC.TGC.CGT.GTA.CC	PGA5
3'TCRAC	ATC.ATA.AAT.TCG.GGT.AGG.ATC.C	PGA5
TCRBV1	AAG.AGA.GAG.CAA.AAG.GAA.ACA.TTC.TTG.AAC	HBVT96
TCRBV2	GCT.CCA.AGG.CCA.CAT.ACG.AGC.AAG.GCG.TCG	MOLT4
TCRBV3	AAA.ATG.AAA.GAA.AAA.GGA.GAT.ATT.CCT.GAG	HBVT22
TCRBV4	CTG.AGG.CCA.CAT.ATG.AGA.GTG.GAT.TTG.TCA	DT110
TCRBV5a	ATA.CTT.CAG.TGA.GAC.ACA.GAG.AAA.C	HBP51
TCRBV5b	TTC.CCT.AAC.TAT.AGC.TCT.GAG.CTG	PL2.5
TCRBV6	CTC.AGG.TGT.GAT.CCA.ATT.TC	HBP04
TCRBV7	ATA.AAT.GAA.AGT.GTG.CCA.AGT.CGC.TTC.TCA	PL4.9
TCRBV8	AAC.GTT.CCG.ATA.GAT.GAT.TCA.GGG.ATG.CCC	YT35
TCRBV9	CAT.TAT.AAA.TGA.AAC.AGT.TCC.AAA.TCG.CTT	PL2.6
TCRBV10	CTT.ATT.CAG.AAA.GCA.GAA.ATA.ATC.AAT.GAG	ATL121
TCRBV11	TCC.ACA.GAG.AAG.GGA.GAT.CTT.TCC.TCT.GAG	PH15
TCRBV12	CTG.AGA.TGT.CAC.CAG.ACT.GAG.AAC.CAC.CGC	HBP54
TCRBV13	CAA.GGA.GAA.GTC.CCC.AAT	HBP34
TCRBV14	GTG.ACT.GAT.AAG.GGA.GAT.GTT.CCT.GAA.GGG	PH21
TCRBV15	GAT.ATA.AAC.AAA.GGA.GAG.ATC.TCT.GAT.GGA	ATL21
TCRBV16	CAT.GAT.AAT.CTT.TAT.CGA.CGT.GTT.ATG.GGA	HBP42
TCRBV17	GCA.CAA.GAA.GCG.ATT.CTC.ATC.TCA.ATG.CCC	HBVT72
TCRBV18	CAT.CTG.TCT.TCT.GGG.GGC.AGG.TCT.CTC.AAA	HBVT56
TCRBV19	ATA.GCT.GAA.GGG.TAC.AGC.GTC.TCT.CGG.GAG	HBVT02
TCRBV20	TCT.AAT.ATT.CAT.CAA.TGG.CCA.GCG.ACC.CT	HUT
TCRBV21	GCA.GTA.GAC.GAT.TCA.CAG.TT	IGRb01
TCRBV22	ATG.CAG.AGC.GAT.AAA.GGA.AG	IGRb03
TCRBV23	ATC.TCA.GAG.AAG.TCT.GAA.AT	IGRb04
TCRBV24	GAT.TTT.AAC.AAT.GAA.GCA.GA	IGRb05
5'TCRBC	CCG.AGG.TCG.CTG.TGT.TTG.AGC.CAT	YT35
3'TCRBC	CTC.TTG.ACC.ATG.GCC.ATC	YT35

Several of the primers have been described previously: 3'TCRAC and 5'TCRAC by Choi et al.[68] TCRAV 2, 3, 5-9, 11, 12 and 17-21 by Oksenberg[69] (17-21 are described as 13-17 in the references); TCRBV 1-5, 7-11, 14-17 by Wucherpfennig et al.[70] The sequences of the TCRBV 20-24 and TCRAV 23-29 family specific oligonucleotide were derived from the DNA sequences of these chains as published by Ferradini et al.[71] and Roman-Roman et al.[72] respectively.

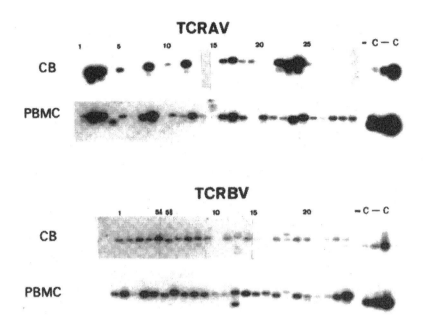

Fig. 2.2. TCRAV and TCRBV repertoires in CB and PBMC. Human fetal tissue was acquired by interruption of pregnancy on non-medical grounds and used for the experiments after informed consent. The gestational age was determined by measurement of the foot length.[73] The use of this material for research purposes was approved by the Ethical Research Committees of the University Hospitals of Leiden and Rotterdam under strict conditions. Adult peripheral blood was obtained from a healthy donor.

(Fig. 2.3, Raaphorst et al.[27]). However, it should be noted that the expression levels of some of the single-member TCR V gene families appeared to be expressed at lower levels in the fetal tissues examined.

Taken together, the diversity of the peripheral TCR V gene repertoire is extensive in early human fetal life since most of the TCR V gene families are already used in TCR rearrangements expressed by fetal T cells.

TCRV-GENE USAGE IN CD4⁺CD8⁻ AND CD4⁻CD8⁺ T-CELL SUBSETS OF HLA IDENTICAL INDIVIDUALS

To determine whether, in addition to MHC, additional genetic factors contribute to the shaping of the mature circulating peripheral T-cell repertoire in humans, we have analyzed the αβ TCR repertoire of four monozygotic twins (Table 2.3; Hawes et al.[20]). As these are genetically identical individuals, it is possible to demonstrate whether the TCRV region gene expression in the peripheral T-cell compartment is determined by inherited factors including the MHC, or whether the expression is shaped in greater part by post-thymic modulations exerted by antigen-driven processes. For these studies, we have determined the relative TCRV gene usage frequencies of the αβ TCR repertoire of the CD4⁺CD8⁻ and CD4⁻CD8⁺ T lymphocyte subsets of monozygotic twins by RT-PCR. The results of the data from the densitometry analyses are shown in Figures 2.4 and 2.5 (Hawes et al.[20]). As can be seen in these figures all pairs of twins demonstrated a striking similarity of the TCRBV and TCRAV repertoires.

Subsequent statistical analysis of the patterns of the TCRV gene usage revealed that the overall usage frequency patterns of TCRBV genes were significantly conserved within a pair of twins. A similar observation was made for the TCRAV patterns, although to a lesser extent than the TCRBV. By determining the correlation values (R^2) of the corresponding TCR V-gene values between twins and unrelated individuals (i.e., unrelated combinations being the comparison of the members of a twin pair to the members of the other three pairs in this panel, thus unrelated individuals), we have seen that there is a higher concordance between the identical individuals, particularly when comparing the TCRBV gene usage. The spread of the R^2 values are shown in Figure 2.6 (Hawes et al.[20]). The R^2 values for the twins were all greater than $R^2 = 0.800$, whereas the unrelated combinations were spread over a wider range that was lower than that of the twins. For the TCRAV usage the R^2 values were also higher between twins compared with unrelated individuals,

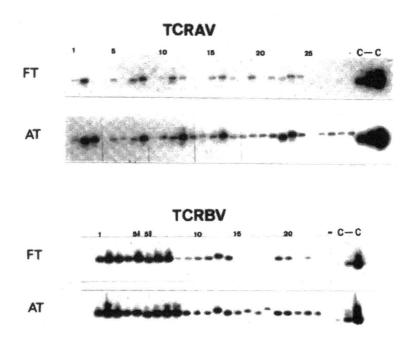

Fig. 2.3. TCRAV and TCRBV repertoires in fetal and pediatric thymi. Post-partum thymi were obtained from pediatric patients undergoing cardiac surgery.

although to a lesser extent than that of the TCRBV gene usage, with the spread of the values being wider and the average being lower.

By comparing multiple individuals exhibiting different levels of HLA-identity and genetic relationship we observed the highest concordance rates in the frequency of TCR V-gene family usage among monozygotic twins and HLA-identical siblings, whereas the concordance rates became gradually smaller when the HLA type and genetic background were diverse (Fig. 2.7). The contribution of the genetic background to the shaping of the circulating repertoires of CD4$^+$CD8$^-$ and CD4$^-$CD8$^+$ T-cell becomes more clear by comparing the relative frequency of usage of individual TCRV gene families within the twins. For instance, the relative amount of TCRBV2 usage compared with TCRBV3 usage is lower in three of the four pairs of twins, but in the other pair (pair 2), both individuals show a much higher frequency of usage of TCRBV2 to that of TCRBV3 (Fig. 2.8). This was seen in both the CD4$^+$CD8$^-$ and CD4$^-$CD8$^+$ subsets for TCRAV and TCRBV families. Similarly, when the usage frequencies of TCR V genes within the CD4$^+$CD8$^-$ and CD4$^-$CD8$^+$ subsets within both members of a twin couple were considered, it became evident that the relative usage frequencies remained consistent within a twin pair but differs among unrelated pairs of twins (Fig. 2.9). For instance, the usage frequency of the TCRBV4 gene family is higher in the CD4$^-$CD8$^+$ subset in three of the four pairs of twins, but is higher in the CD4$^+$CD8$^-$ in the other pair (pair 3). We have noticed this phenomenon in our twin

Table 2.3. Dates of birth (d.o.b.) and HLA types of the monozygotic twins examined

Twin Pairs	d.o.b.	HLA-type Class I	Class II
FN/NN	04/24/64	A1, A3 B7, B8 Cw7	DR2, DR3
PG/JG	11/19/65	A1, A2 B8, B44 Cw5, Cw7	DR3, DR5
TKG/JNG	02/11/60	A3, A31 B60 Cw3, Cw10	DR4, DR11
AN/AL	05/19/76	A2 B57, B60 Cw3, Cw6	DR6, DR7

All four pairs are natives of The Netherlands and therefore have been exposed to the same regional environmental antigens, but were born over a time period in which they were subsequently subject to varying childhood vaccination protocols.

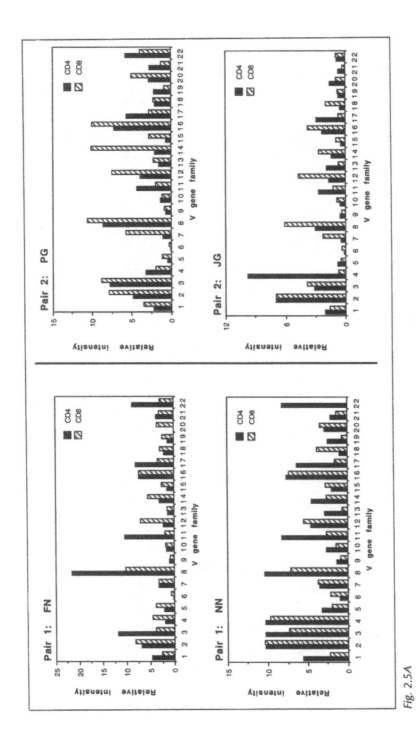

Fig. 2.5A

Fig. 2.4. The complete TCRBV region gene usage patterns in the CD4+ and CD8+ T lymphocyte subsets of monozygotic twins determined by PCR: The values were determined by measuring the relative intensity by densitometry of the autoradiograms from Southern blots of the PCR products. Reprinted from Hawes et al. J Immunol 1993; 150:2033-2045; © 1992, The Journal of Immunology.

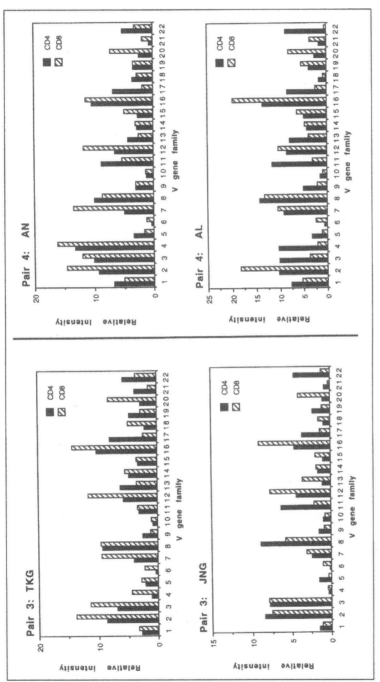

Fig. 2.5B

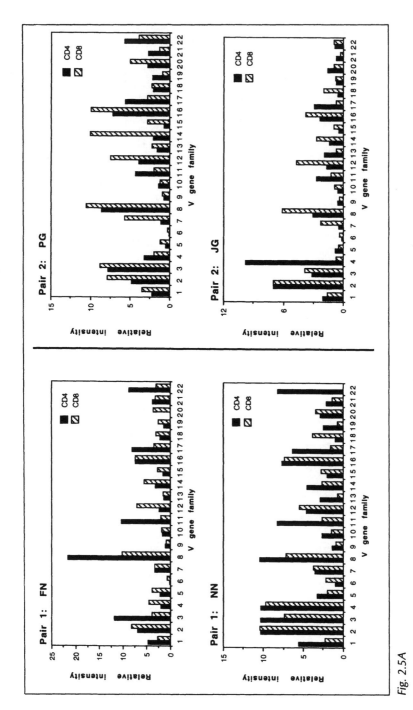

Fig. 2.5A

Fig. 2.5. The complete TCRAV region gene usage patterns in the CD4+ and CD8+ T lymphocyte subsets of monozygotic twins determined by PCR. The values were determined by measuring the relative intensity by densitometry of the autoradiograms from Southern blots of the PCR products. Reprinted from Hawes et al. J Immunol 1993; 150:2033-2045; ©1992, The Journal of Immunology.

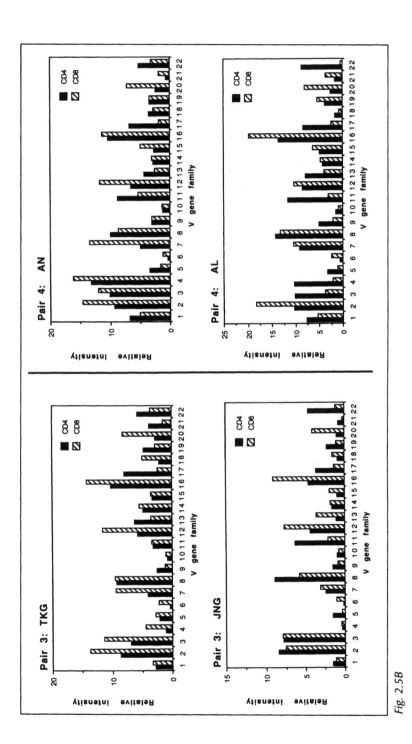

Fig. 2.5B

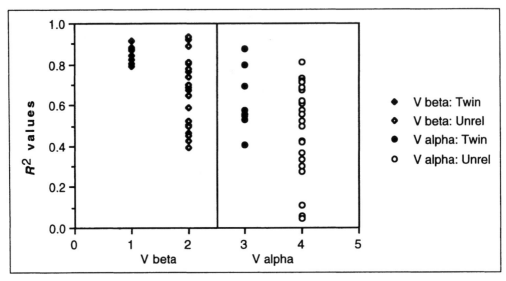

Fig. 2.6.The distribution of the correlation values (R^2) of the αβTCR V gene usage patterns are represented for the comparisons between monozygotic twins (solid symbols) and unrelated combinations (open symbols). As seen by the distribution of the values for the twins compared to that of the unrelated combinations, the twins show a higher level of concordance, particularly for the Vβ where all the values are > 0.800 (R^2 = 1.000 being a perfect correlation and R^2 = 0.000 being no correlation). The Vα correlation is also higher between twins than unrelated individuals, albeit to a lesser extent than that of the Vβ. Reprinted from Hawes et al. J Immunol 1993; 150:2033-2045, © 1992, The Journal of Immunology.

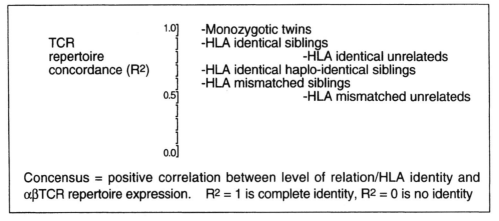

Fig. 2.7. Concordance in peripheral αβTCR repertoire: Comparisons between HLA identical/non-identical, related and unrelated individuals.

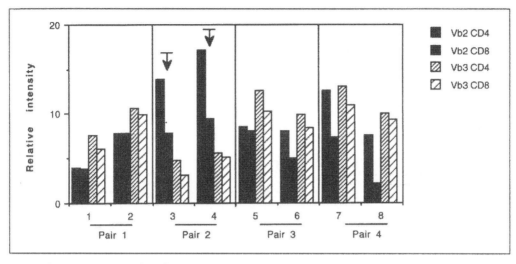

Fig. 2.8. The conservation of the relative V region gene frequency pattern within a pair of monozygotic twins represented by the relative frequency of Vβ2 and Vβ3 of the CD4⁺ and CD8⁺ subsets. Pair 2 demonstrates the twin specific usage frequency: Both individuals share the higher usage of Vβ2 to that of Vβ3, whereas in the other 3 pairs the converse is true. Reprinted from Hawes et al. J Immunol 1993; 150:2033-2045, © 1992, The Journal of Immunology.

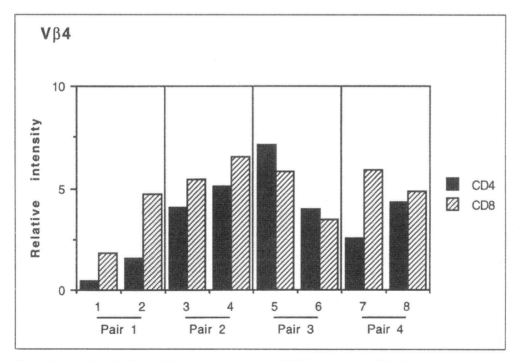

Fig. 2.9. Example of pair specific skewing where the TCRV gene usage differs between the pairs of monozygotic twins, but is conserved within a set of twins. This is represented here by TCRBV4, which is skewed to the CD8⁺ subset within both members of the twins pairs 1, 2 and 4, whereas within pair 3 the skewing is to the CD4⁺ subset.

panel also for the usage frequencies of the TCRBV2, 5, 6, 8, 19 and TCRAV7, 16, 18 and 21 gene families. In these cases, the TCRV gene family is skewed either to the CD4⁺CD8⁻ or CD4⁻CD8⁺ subset or is represented in equal amounts. These conserved TCRV gene usage frequencies patterns within sets of twins suggests a selection bias predominantly based on genetic factors.

DISTRIBUTION OF TCRV GENES IN THE CD4⁺CD8⁻ AND CD4⁻CD8⁺ SUBSETS

To address the question whether the TCRV region genes are equally distributed between the CD4⁺CD8⁻ and CD4⁻CD8⁺ T-cell subsets, or if preferential skewing could be detected, the relative usage frequencies of each individual TCRAV and TCRBV gene family between the subsets were examined. The R^2 correlation between the CD4⁺CD8⁻and CD4⁻CD8⁺ subsets was lower in all cases (TCRBV R^2 = 0.505 to 0.795, mean = 0.674; TCRAV R^2 = 0.138 to 0.573, mean = 0.399) than the R^2 values between the corresponding subsets within the twins, indicating that there were indeed differences in the distribution of at least some of the TCRV gene families between the CD4⁺CD8⁻ and CD4⁻CD8⁺ subsets within each twin pair. Using the paired sample Student's t-test we found that, within the majority of individuals studied (n = 8), a significant preferential skewing of several of the TCRAV and TCRBV gene segments to either the CD4⁺CD8⁻or CD4⁻CD8⁺ subset exists, apparently regardless of the genetic background of the individuals. In Figure 2.10 examples of such CD4⁺CD8⁻ or CD4⁻CD8⁺ skewing patterns are shown. As listed in Table 2.4, within the CD4⁺CD8⁻ subset the usage frequencies of the TCRAV 11, 17, 22 and TCRBV 3, 9, 12, 18 gene segments were significantly increased; and within the CD4⁻CD8⁺ subset, the TCRAV 2, 6, 12, 15, 20 and TCRBV 7, 14, 17 frequencies were significantly enhanced, with probability values ranging from p = 0.0476 to < 0.001.

NON-RANDOM EMPLOYMENT OF TCRBV6 AND TCRBJ ELEMENTS IN TCR β-CHAIN REARRANGEMENTS

In order to study in more detail the generation of diversity of the human peripheral TCR repertoire during development, we have analyzed TCR β chain rearrangements employing a TCRBV element belonging to the multi-member TCRBV6 family by DNA sequencing. Material was obtained from an 11, 13 and 17 week old fetus which included cord blood, spleen, bone marrow, liver and thymus. The fetal sequences were compared with adult TCR β chain rearrangements, which were obtained from spleen (AS), from post-partum thymus (AT), and from PBMC (APBMC).

The usage of TCRBV6 gene elements in TCR β chain rearrangements present in fetal cord blood and adult peripheral blood was skewed to a number of the 14 currently identified TCRBV6 elements. As shown in Figure 2.11, we were unable to detect rearrangement of the

TCRBV6S2, TCRBV6S5 and TCRBV6S7b in either fetal cord blood or adult peripheral blood, whereas the other TCRBV6 family members could be found at various frequencies. Similar analyses in fetal liver, spleen and bone marrow and in adult spleen and thymus revealed a similar pattern of expression of the various TCRBV6 elements (not shown, see Raaphorst et al.[22]).

The employment of the TCRBJ gene elements in TCR β chain rearrangements using a TCRBV6 gene family member showed that in the 11 week old fetus, approximately 90% of the TCR rearrangements employed a TCRBJ2 element, independently of the tissue of origin (Fig. 2.12, only FCB and APBMC are shown; Raaphorst et al.[22]). In fetal tissues obtained at 13 and 17 weeks of gestation, and in the adult tissues, TCRBJ1 elements were used at higher frequencies (20-40%). Within the fetal and adult rearrangements employing a TCRBJ2 element, an overall high frequency of usage of the TCRBJ2S1 and TCRBJ2S7 elements was noted. In general, TCRBJ2S1 was used at comparable levels in fetal and adult rearrangements, whereas the usage frequency of the TCRBJ2S7 element suggested an increase with age in the majority of tissues analyzed (25% in the 11 week old fetus, 30% in the 13 week old fetus, and 50% in adult spleen and APBMC). Also, several TCRBJ elements (most notably TCRBJ1S3, TCRBJ1S4, TCRBJ2S4 and TCRBJ2S6) were infrequently encountered in both fetal and adult rearrangements.

Taken together, these analyses revealed that the various germ-line encoded elements which make up the TCR β chains are not randomly employed both in fetal and adult TCR β chain rearrangements.

GENERATION OF CDR3-DIVERSITY: COMPOSITION OF THE N_1-D-N_2 SEGMENT OF THE CDR3 REGION OF TCR β-CHAINS EXPRESSING MEMBERS OF THE TCRBV6 GENE FAMILY

To investigate the generation of CDR3 diversity in great detail, we have examined the contribution of the TCRBD elements and N-nucleotides in the make-up of the CDR3 regions. In general, the employment of the TCRBD1 and TCRBD2 gene elements was roughly comparable in fetal and adult TCR β chain rearrangements containing an identifiable D element (data not shown). The presence and length of N-regions in the TCR β chain rearrangements showed an age-dependent distribution, which was most clearly illustrated by the number of sequences lacking N-regions or containing only one N-nucleotide. As shown in Figure 2.13 the majority of the TCR rearrangements obtained from cord blood of the 11 and 13 week old fetuses contained one or no N-nucleotide in the CDR3 region. Within these rearrangements, the distribution pattern of N-regions did not significantly differ in sequences obtained from haematopoietic organs (liver, bone marrow) or from the periphery (spleen) (not shown, Raaphorst et al.[22]). None of the N-regions detected in cord blood of the 11 and 13 week old fetuses were longer than nine nucleotides, whereas TCR β chain rearrangements derived from adult peripheral blood exhibited longer N-regions even up to 22 nucleotides in length. Less than 5% of the sequences derived from APBMC and spleen contained one or no detectable N-nucleotide. Fetal TCR β chain CDR3 regions obtained at 11 and 13 weeks of gestation were generally smaller than adult TCR β chain CDR3 regions: 64% of the combined TCR β chain rearrangements at 11 weeks and 47% of the combined rearrangements at 13 weeks of gestation encompassed a CDR3 region consisting of seven nucleotides or less. In APBMC and adult spleen, these values were 33 and 14% respectively. This limited CDR3 diversity on the basis of numbers of N-nucleotide additions in fetal tissue or thymocytes compared to adult thymocytes or T lymphocytes has also been noted by others (see Krangel et al.[28]; George et al.[29]; Bonati et al.[30]).

Amino Acid Composition
of Fetal and Adult TCR β Chain CDR3 Regions

Analysis of the amino acid composition of the CDR3 regions in the TCR β chains revealed that all three reading frames (RFs) of the TCRDB elements were used without clear preference for a particular RF. This is illustrated by the amino acid composition of CDR3 regions determined in productive TCR β chain rearrangements cloned

Table 2.4. Statistical analysis of skewing of the αβTCR V region genes within the CD4⁺ and CD8⁺ subsets

V gene	Mean CD4-CD8	Paired t value	P-value (2-tail)
Vα2	-2.770	-2.463	0.0433
Vα6	-0.914	-4.070	0.0047
Vα11	4.193	3.778	0.0069
Vα12	-3.585	-5.986	< 0.001
Vα15	-1.176	-4.421	0.0031
Vα17	4.120	7.851	< 0.001
Vα20	-3.067	-3.900	0.0059
Vα22	3.922	3.609	0.0086
Vβ3	1.345	5.584	< 0.001
Vβ7	-1.231	-2.398	0.0476
Vβ9	1.648	2.789	0.0269
Vβ12	1.742	4.377	0.0032
Vβ14	-3.206	-4.974	0.0016
Vβ17	-0.754	-3.337	0.0125
Vβ18	1.934	4.194	0.0041

The P-values for the skewing between the CD4⁺ and CD8⁺ subsets are calculated by the two-tailed paired t-test of the normalized densitometry data. The positive values for the paired t value indicate skewing to the CD4⁺ subset and the negative values indicate skewing to the CD8⁺ subset. Reprinted from Hawes et al. J Immunol 1993; 150:2033-2045, © 1992, The Journal of Immunology.

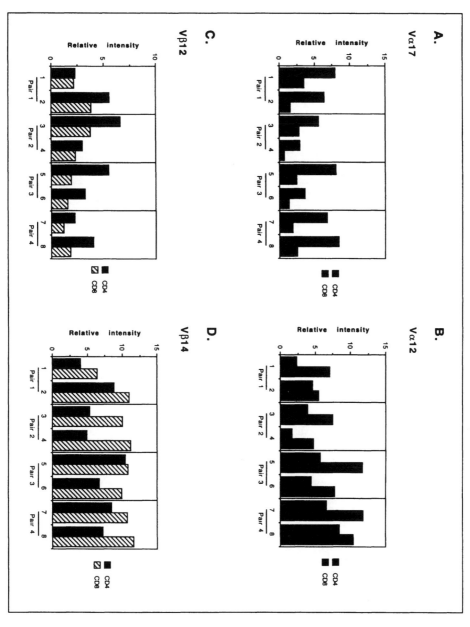

Fig. 2.10. Examples of the skewing patterns of the αβTCR V region genes to the CD4+ and CD8+: 2.10a and 2.10b represent significant skewing to the CD4+ and CD8+ subsets respectively for TCRAV gene families. (P-values = < 0.001) 2.10c and 210d represent significant skewing to the CD4+ and CD8+ subsets respectively for TCRBV gene families (P-values = < 0.004).

from FCB11, FCB13, and APBMC (Fig. 2.14); similar observations were made for the recombinations cloned from the other fetal and adult tissues. In general, the usage frequencies of amino acids encoded by the CDR3 region of both fetal as well as adult TCR β chain rearrangements revealed a non-random distribution pattern. For instance A, R, G, S and T residues were used at high frequencies, whereas N, C, H, I, K, M and Y were not present or used at low frequencies. These patterns of amino acid distribution were similar in both fetal and adult rearrangements and exhibited no organ dependency (see Raaphorst et al.[22]).

INDIVIDUAL SPECIFIC AMINO ACID MOTIFS ARE DISCERNIBLE IN CDR3 REGIONS OF TCR β CHAIN REARRANGEMENTS

Scrutiny of N_1-D-N_2 region sequences derived from different TCRBV genes of four donors revealed that particular amino acid sequence motifs were found. These motifs were comprised of N-nucleotide sequences and exhibited individual specific characteristics. This finding suggests that the makeup of CDR3 region N-nucleotide sequences during the recombination process of TCR β chain sequences does not seem to occur in an apparent random fashion (Table 2.5). The composition of the CDR3 region seems to be in part based on individual specific usage of particular amino acids, resulting in the incorporation of amino acid motifs independent of the employment of TCRBV genes.

2.3 DISCUSSION

Little is known about the mechanisms controlling the shaping of the mature peripheral T-cell repertoire. In humans, it is unclear whether the repertoire is randomly expressed, extensively modified by exposure to environmental antigens, or under the influence of genetic predetermination. Most of our current knowledge is derived from studies in mice. There, genetic influences are apparent in inbred strains of mice.[31] In the example of superantigens such as Mls and staphylococcal enterotoxins, certain strains of mice expressing a particular haplotype and endogenous superantigen show a complete deletion of various TCRV elements that are reactive against these superantigens.[32,33] For instance, mice of the Mls-1ᵃ type have deleted TCRBV 6, 7, 8.1, and 9 regions.[34] As of yet, this complete deletion of an entire TCRV gene family has not been observed in humans. Further genetic influences in mice have been apparent such as the reported skewing of various TCRV genes to either the CD4⁺CD8⁻ and CD4⁻CD8⁺ subset.[35-37] It is likely that this has not been so readily apparent in humans because of the fact that humans are outbred and therefore more polymorphic compared with mice.

In a number of experiments aimed to analyze the usage patterns of TCRAV and TCRBV families by T cells in PBMC of adult donors, it became clear that all of the TCRV gene families identified to date were detectable.[17,20,38-44] In general, major deletions or

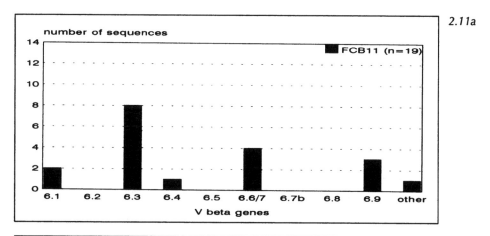

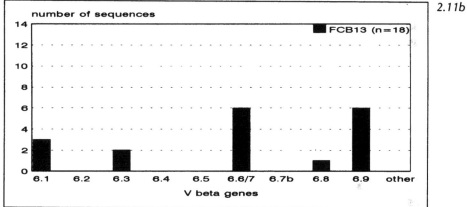

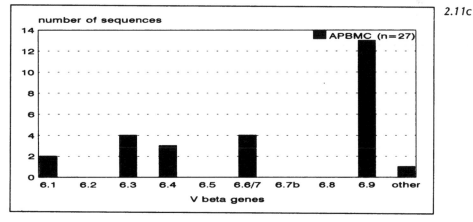

Fig. 2.11. TCRBV6 usage frequencies in FCB and APBMC. To identify the DNA sequence of the TCRBV6 regions, the PCR products were gel-purified after 30 cycles and reamplified for 15 cycles of PCR using Magic PCR-preps™ DNA Purification System (Promega Corp., Madison, WI, U.S.A.). These PCR-products were blunt-ended and ligated into pUC19 Sma I digested vector the nucleotide sequence was determined using the ⊤7sequencing™ kit (Pharmacia, Uppsala, Sweden) following the instructions of the manufacturer.

Fig. 2.12. TCRBJ usage
frequencies in FCB and
APBMC.

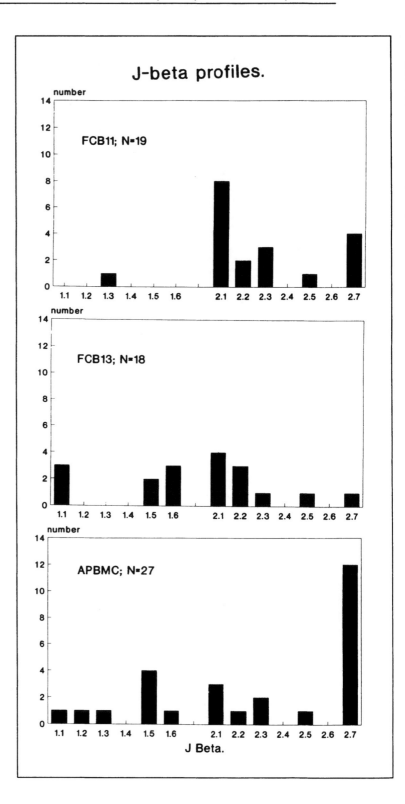

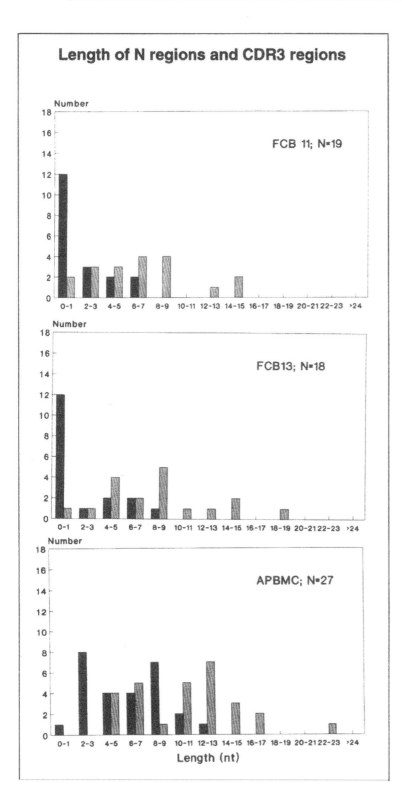

Fig. 2.13. Size of N-regions (black bars) and CDR3 regions (shaded bars; the D-element + flanking N regions) in human FCB and APBMC TCR β chain rearrangements.

compressions of the TCRAV and TCRBV repertoires at the family level are not apparent in humans. Furthermore, the usage patterns of TCRAV and TCRBV gene families were subject to individual specific variations.

Several studies have provided evidence that in humans the composition of the mature T-cell compartment is considerably influenced by genetic factors which include factors which are directly involved in the interactions between MHC molecules and peptide and the TCR during thymic maturation.[45-49] This conclusion is also derived from the observation that the overall patterns of gene usage frequency and skewing to the CD4+CD8- and CD4-CD8+ subsets of both individuals in a pair of identical twins are far more similar to each other than when comparing unrelated individuals.[20] Differences observed within the pairs of twins were anticipated because it is impossible to control for the immune status of the individuals at the time of blood

Table 2.5. Conserved amino acid motifs in the N-D-N region of TCRBV5S1/5S4, TCRBV11 and TCRBV14 genes derived from PBMC of four donors

Donors

A
TCRBV5	DGGI
TCRBV11	DGGI
TCRBV5	VGT
TCRBV11	GTV

B
TCRBV5	GQGG
TCRBV11	GGLG
TCRBV14	GTGG
TCRBV5	PGQ
TCRBV14	PGQ

C
TCRBV5	AGG, AG, AGTG, LAGGG
TCRBV11	ATG
TCRBV14	LAGVG
TCRBV11	SRA
TCRBV14	SRA

D
TCRBV5	SNRDR
TCRBV11	RLN, RGSN, GRS, RSS
TCRBV14	RNNRG, NRGGNS
TCRBV5	VGG
TCRBV11	VGG

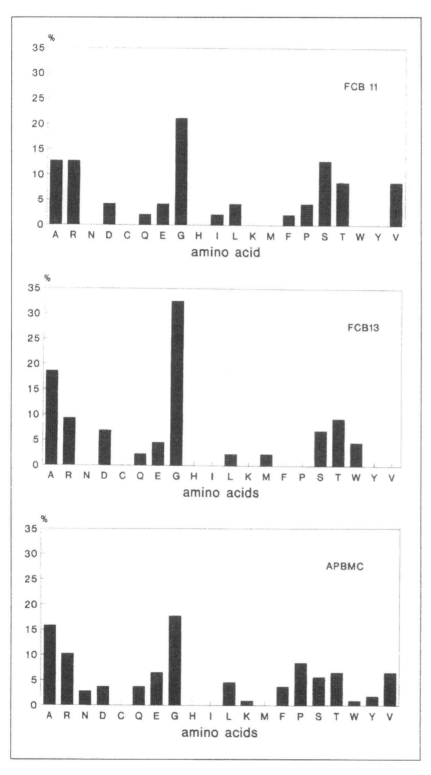

Fig. 2.14. Usage frequencies of amino acids in TCR β chain CDR3 regions. (Reprinted with permission from Raaphorst et al. Int. Imm. 1994; 6:1-9).

donation, and the fact that they are mature individuals resulting in variable exposure to environmental antigens. Taking these factors into consideration, such similarities as we have observed in TCRV gene usage are even more remarkable, suggesting that the repertoire available remains fairly stable in the periphery of these adults even after exposure to environmental antigens and post-thymic modulations, which can influence the expression patterns of the αβ TCR in the mature repertoire.

The evident skewing of several TCRV regions to either the CD4⁺CD8⁻ or CD4⁻CD8⁺ subset which was consistent in the majority of cases is a phenomenon that has been demonstrated in mice, and more recently, in humans.[21,50] These reports are consistent with our findings in the skewing of TCRBV14, TCRBV18,[21] and TCRAV12.[51] This is suggestive of these particular TCRV region gene products having a preferential interaction (or selective advantage) with MHC class II molecules (for skewing to the CD4⁺CD8⁻ subset) and MHC class I molecules (for skewing to the CD4⁻CD8⁺ subset) in the process of positive selection during thymic maturation, regardless of the populations chosen for study. Also it has been reported that TCRBV5S1 and TCRBV6S7 are skewed to the CD4⁺CD8⁻ subset and TCRAV2S3 (in some cases) to the CD4⁻CD8⁺ subset as determined by mAb.[21,45] This observation is also in agreement with our findings as we have also screened our panel of twins with the αβTCRV region mAb (not shown, Hawes et al.[20]). However, it should be taken into consideration when making comparisons between mAb data and the PCR method of analysis that skewing of individual members of a TCR V gene family (such as for instance TCRBV6S7) can remain unnoted, particularly when the mAb recognizes only one member of the TCRV gene family and the oligonucleotide PCR primer is designed to amplify multiple members of a family of TCRV gene products.

Although it is unlikely that this skewing is caused by negative selection (depletion) from the reciprocal subset, the possibility does remain that a single member of a TCRV gene family has been negatively selected in these individuals, but this would go undetected, particularly in the TCRV gene families that contain several members, inasmuch as the oligonucleotide primers used are family-specific detecting multiple family members and the deletion of one member within a family could not be readily discriminated.

Further confirming the genetic predisposition for a given αβ TCR repertoire is the fact that several skewing patterns were represented in a pair-specific manner. When examining genetically nonidentical individuals, this pattern would either be overlooked as being insignificant in skewing as exemplified in Figure 2.9, when within one set of twins the TCRV gene is skewed to the CD4⁺CD8⁻ subset, whereas, in another set, it is skewed to the CD4⁻CD8⁺ subset (as with TCRBV4, 6, 19 and TCRAV18, 21; p-values = 0.0787 to 0.4834);

or would be considered as significant skewing to the subsets in the majority of the population (as seen with TCRBV2, 5, 8 and TCRAV7, 16; p-values = 0.0363 to < 0.001). This would be the case in this study if we had only one member of each twin pair for comparison. This presents evidence that the shape of the overall repertoire available is dependent on genetic factors such as thymic MHC expression and subsequent selection. It is also possible that this "pair-specific" skewing phenomenon would be seen with the rest of the TCRV families we now describe as significant skewing regardless of genetic background if a larger panel of individuals were examined. Recently, other groups have also reported a higher similarity of TCRV gene usage between twins and HLA identical siblings,[52] and correlations are becoming apparent between HLA-haplotype and the skewing of TCRV-genes within the CD4+CD8- or CD4-CD8+ subsets among HLA identical siblings.[47,53]

We have also observed in our studies that the relative usage frequencies of individual TCRV-gene families remains consistent between the twins. It should be noted here that a greater consistency between twins was observed in the TCRBV gene usage compared with the TCRAV. Because we have discounted the possibility that this is caused by the lack of repeatability of the PCR with the TCRAV primer set, this is consistent with the postulation that the TCRAV chain is mainly concerned with the recognition and binding to foreign antigen[51] which would explain the greater diversity seen in this study for the TCRAV genes. The expression of the TCRAV chain genes in the mature periphery could therefore be influenced to a greater extent by post-thymic modulations and foreign antigen exposure, which would assure greater diversity in the specificity for foreign antigen peptides; whereas the TCRBV gene usage may be more important in acquiring the restriction to self-MHC molecules that then would be selected for specific interactions with MHC in the thymic microenvironment.[54]

Our studies have also demonstrated that the distribution of TCRBV elements in fetal TCR β rearrangements using the multi-member TCRBV6 family was non-random. However, although the adult TCRBV repertoire is thought to be more diverse than the fetal TCRBV repertoire, adult TCRBV6 rearrangements also exhibited a similar pattern of non-random usage of TCRBV6 genes. As it has been shown that the expression pattern of human TCRV elements does not correlate with their chromosomal position,[55] it is unlikely that preferential employment of particular TCRBV6 elements can be explained by the organization of the TCR β chain locus. Furthermore, although several pseudogenes have been described in the TCRBV6 family,[56,57] all TCRBV6 genes detected in this study have previously been detected in functional TCR rearrangements. As TCRBV6 profiles were similar in hematopoietic organs and peripheral organs, a possible explanation for the non-random patterns of TCRBV gene usage may be variation in the activities of the promoters of the various TCRBV6 elements.[56]

We also showed that usage of TCRBJ elements in fetal TCR β chain rearrangements was non-random. In contrast to mouse fetal TCR β chain rearrangements, where TCRBJ1 and TCRBJ2 elements are used at equal frequencies,[58] early human fetal TCR β chain sequences primarily used TCRBJ2 elements. The usage pattern of TCRBJ elements remained skewed towards TCRBJ2 elements in adult life, which has also been reported in several other studies.[15,17,18,23] The high frequency of usage of TCRBJ2 elements, particularly in the 11 week old fetal tissues, can be related to the TCR β chain enhancer located 3' of TCRBC2 which may influence their accessibility to the recombinase machinery.[59-61] Alternatively, as the TCRBD1 element can recombine to both TCRBJ1 and TCRBJ2 elements and secondary rearrangements are possible, TCRBJ2 segments are more likely to be used in TCR β chain rearrangements. Indeed, within the sequences containing an identifiable TCRBD element, 17% of the fetal rearrangements and 21% of the adult rearrangements constituted a TCRBD1-TCRBJ2 recombination (data not shown).

The high frequency of usage of TCRBJ2S1 and TCRBJ2S7 (and the low expression of the TCRBJ2S4 and TCRBJ2S6 elements) has been described in the majority of the adult peripheral TCR β repertoires examined to date.[15,17,18,23,24] We showed that these TCRBJ usage profiles are already discernible in early fetal TCR β chain rearrangements obtained from hematopoietic and peripheral tissues. Although expression of TCRBJ elements can be influenced by selection of rearrangements,[62] several recent publications show that the situation is more complex. Firstly, the TCRBJ usage patterns of both mouse and human TCRBD-TCRBJ transcripts, which were unexpressed and therefore unselected, were found to be similar to the TCRBJ profile of completed TCRBV-D-J rearrangements.[17,63] Also, analysis of the TCRBJ usage patterns of human TCR rearrangements cloned from antigen-selected T cells[64-66] showed that the usage of TCRBJ elements was similar to that of unselected peripheral TCR recombinations. Taken together, these observations suggest that the unselected TCRBJ repertoire as found in hematopoietic tissues is similar to the unselected peripheral TCRBJ repertoire and that of selected, antigen-specific peripheral T cells. Therefore, the human peripheral TCRBJ repertoire seems generally a reflection of rearrangement frequencies of J elements.

We have demonstrated that the development of the mature peripheral αβ TCR repertoire is not a completely random process in man, but rather reveals a genetic predisposition to a certain pattern of expression in a given individual. It is tempting to speculate on the mechanisms controlling the shaping of the TCR repertoire and the effects of positive and negative selection during thymic maturation as a consequence of self peptide/MHC interactions, and moreover, the bearing this has on the examination of the TCR in response to (self) antigen in disease states. Furthermore, although the potential TCR αβ repertoire is estimated to be of a size of at least 10^{15} TCR specificities, based on random employment of TCRV, D and J elements and the contribution of the junctional diversity,[3,7,8,15] we and others have shown that usage of TCRBV and TCRBJ elements in human adult TCRβ chain rearrangements and the usage of amino acids in the antigen binding regions are non-random. Therefore, the actual adult TCRβ repertoires in the circulation are seemingly smaller than estimated on the basis of stochastic usage of TCRV, D and J elements.

ACKNOWLEDGEMENTS

This research was supported by the "Nationaal Reumafonds" of the Netherlands (Grant 90/NR/276), the Macropa Foundation and the J.A. Cohen Institute for Radio-Pathology and Radiation Protection (IRS).

REFERENCES

1. Marrack P, Kappler J. The T-cell receptor. Science 1987; 238:1073-79.
2. Bjorkman PJ, Saper MA, Samraoi B et al. Structure of the human class I histocompatibility antigen HLA-A2. Nature 1987; 329:506-12.
3. Davis MM, Bjorkman PJ. T-cell antigen receptor genes and T-cell recognition. Nature 1988; 334:395-402.
4. Strominger JL. Developmental biology of T-cell receptors. Science 1989; 244:943-50.
5. Meuer SC, Acuto O, Hercend T et al. The human T-cell receptor. Annu Rev Immunol 1984; 2:23-50.
6. Clevers H, Alarcon B, Wileman T et al. The T-cell receptor/CD3 complex: a dynamic protein assemble. Annu Rev Immunol 1988; 6:629-62.
7. Kronenberg M, Siu G, Hood L et al. The molecular genetics of the T-cell antigen receptor and T-cell antigen recognition. Ann Rev Immunol 1986; 4:529-91.
8. Seboun E, Robinson MA, Kindt TJ et al. Insertion/deletion-related polymorphisms in human T-cell receptor β gene complex. J Exp Med 1989; 170:1263-70.
9. Lafaille JJ, DeCloux A, Bonneville M et al. Junctional sequences of T-cell receptor gamma delta genes: implications for gamma delta T-cell lineages and for novel intermediate of V-(D)-J joining. Cell 1989; 59:859-70.
10. Novotny J, Tonegawa S, Saito H et al. Secondary, tertiary and quarternary structure of T-cell-specific-immunoglobulin-like polypeptide chains. Proc Natl Acad Sci 1986; 83:742-46.
11. Bougueleret L, Claverie J-M. Variability analysis of the human and mouse T-cell receptor β chains. Immunogenetics 1987; 26:304-08.
12. Chothia C, Boswell DR, Lesk AM. The outline structure of the T-cell αβ receptor. EMBO J 1988; 7:3745-55.
13. Claverie JM, Prochnicka-Chalufour A, Bougueleret L. Implications of a Fab-like structure for the T-cell receptor. Immunol Today 1989; 10:10-14.
14. Chien Y, Davis MM. How αβ T-cell receptors 'see' peptide/MHC complexes. Immunol Today 1993; 14:597-602.

15. Moss PAH, Rosenberg WMC, Bell JI. The human T-cell receptor in health and disease. Annu Rev Immunol 1992; 10:71-96.

16. Moss PAH, Rosenberg WMC, Zintzaras E et al. Characterization of the human T-cell receptor α-chain repertoire and demonstration of a genetic influence on Vα usage. Eur J Immunol 1993; 23:1153-59.

17. Rosenberg WMC, Moss PAH, Bell JI. Variation in human T-cell receptor Vβ and Jβ repertoire: analysis using anchor polymerase chain reaction. Eur J Immunol 1992; 22:541-49.

18. Robinson MA. Usage of human T-cell receptor Vβ, Jβ,Cβ and Vα gene segments is not proportional to gene number. Hum Immunol 1992; 35:60-67.

19. Akolkar PN, Gulwani-Alkokar B, Pergolizzi R et al. Influence of HLA genes on T-cell receptor V segment frequencies and expression levels in peripheral blood lymphocytes. J Immunol 1993; 150:2761-73.

20. Hawes GE, Struyk L, Van den Elsen PJ. Differential usage of T-cell receptor V gene segments in CD4+ and CD8+ subsets of T lymphocytes in monozygotic twins. J Immunol 1993; 150:2033-45.

21. Davey MP, Meyer MM, Munkirs M et al. T-cell receptor variable β genes show differential expression in CD4+ and CD8+ cells. Hum Immunol 1991; 32:194-202.

22. Raaphorst FM, Kaijzel EL, Van Tol MJD et al. Non-random employment of Vβ6 and Jβ gene elements and conserved amino acid usage profiles in CDR3 regions of human fetal and adult TCR β chain rearrangements. Int Immunol 1994; 6:1-9.

23. Grunewald J, Jeddi-Tehrani M, Pisa E et al. Analysis of Jβ gene segment usage by CD4+ and CD8+ human peripheral blood T lymphocytes. Int Immunol 1992; 4:643-50.

24. Jeddi-Tehrani M, Grunewald J, Hodara V et al. Nonrandom T-cell receptor Jβ usage pattern in human CD4+ and CD8+ peripheral T cells. Hum Immunol 1994; 40:93-100.

25. Saito T, Sussman JI, Ashwell JD et al. Marked differences in the efficiency of expression of distinct αβ T-cell receptor heterodimers. J Immunol 1989; 143:3379-84.

26. Robinson MA, Mitchell MP, Wei S et al. Organization of human T-cell receptor β-chain genes: clusters of Vβ genes are present on chromosomes 7 and 9. Proc Natl Acad Sci 1993; 90:2433-37.

27. Raaphorst FM, Van Bergen J, Langlois van den Bergh et al. Usage of TCRAV and TCRVB gene families in human fetal and adult TCR rearrangements. Immunogenetics 1994; 39:343-50.

28. Krangel MS, Yssel H, Brocklehurst C et al. A distinct wave of human γ/δ lymphocytes in the early fetal thymus: evidence for controlled gene rearrangement and cytokine production. J Exp Med 1990; 172:847-59.

29. George JF, Schroeder HW. Developmental regulation of Dβ reading frame and junctional diversity in T-cell receptor-β transcripts from human thymus. J Immunol 1992; 148:1230-39.

30. Bonati A, Zanelli P, Ferrari S et al. T-cell receptor β chain gene rearrangement and expression during human thymic ontogenesis. Blood 1992; 79:1472-83.

31. Vacchio MS, Hodes RJ. Selective decreases in T-cell receptor Vβ expression: decreased expression of specific Vβ families is associated with expression of multiple MHC and non-MHC gene products. J Exp Med 1989; 170:1335-46.

32. Gao E-K, Kanagawa O, Sprent J. Capacity of unprimed CD4+ and CD8+ T cells expressing Vβ11⁻ receptors to respond to I-E alloantigens in vivo. J Exp Med 1989; 170:1947-57.

33. Liao N-S, Maltzman J, Raulet DH. Positive selection determines T-cell receptor Vβ14 usage by CD8+ cells. J Exp Med 1989; 170:135-43.

34. Acha-Orbea H, Palmer E. Mls: a retrovirus exploits the immune system. Immunol Today 1991; 12:356-61.

35. Utsunomiya Y, Bill J, Palmer E et al. Analysis of a monoclonal rat antibody directed to the α-chain variable region (Vα3) of the mouse T-cell antigen receptor. J Immunol 1989; 143:2602-08.

36. Liao N-S, Maltzman J, Raulet D. Expression of the Vβ5.1 gene by murine peripheral T cells is controlled by MHC genes and skewed to the CD8+ subset. J Immunol 1990; 144:844-48.

37. Jameson SC, Kaye J, Gascoigne NRJ. A T-cell receptor Vα region selectively expressed in CD4+ cells. J Immunol 1990; 145:1324-31.

38. Doherty PJ, Roifman CM, Pan S et al. Expression of the human T-cell receptor Vβ repertoire. Mol Immunol 1991; 6:607-12.

39. Genevée C, Diu A, Nierat J et al. An experimentally validated panel of subfamily-specific oligonucleotide primers (Vα1-w29/Vβ1-w24) for the study of human T-cell receptor variable V gene segment usage by polymerase chain reaction. Eur J Immunol 1992; 22:1261-69.

40. Hu H, Queirò MR, Tilanus MGJ, de Weger RA et al. Expression of T-cell receptor α and β variable genes in normal and malignant human T cells. Br J Hematol 1993; 84:39-48.

41. Malhorta U, Spielman R, Concannon P. Variability in T-cell receptor Vβ gene usage in human peripheral blood lymphocytes. Studies of identical twins, siblings, and insulin-dependent diabetes mellitus patients. J Immunol 1992; 149:1802-08.

42. Dave VP, Larché M, Rencher SD et al. Restricted usage of T-cell receptor Va sequence and variable-joining pairs after normal T-cell development and bone marrow transplantation. Hum Immunol 1993; 37:178-84.

43. Geursen A, Skinner MA, Townsend LA et al. Population study of T-cell receptor Vβ gene usage in peripheral blood lymphocytes: differences in ethnic groups. Clin Exp Immunol 1993; 94:201-07.

44. Hu HZ, de Weger RA, Bosboom-Kalsbeek K et al. T-cell receptor Vβ variable gene family expression in human peripheral blood lymphocytes at the mRNA and membrane protein level. Clin Exp Immunol 1992; 88:335-40.

45. Genevée C, Farace F, Chung V et al. Influence of human leukocyte antigen genes on TCR V gene segment frequencies. Int Immunol 1994; 6(10):1497-1504.

46. Reed EF, Tugulea SL and Suciu-foca N. Influence of HLA class I and class II antigens on the peripheral T-cell receptor repertoire. Hum Immunol 1994; 40:111-22.

47. Gulwani-Akolkar B, Posnett D.N, Janson C.H et al. T-cell receptor V segment frequencies in peripheral blood T cells correlate with human leukocyte antigen type. J Exp Med 1991; 174:1139-46.

48. Utz U, Biddison WE, McFarland HF et al. Skewed T-cell receptor repertoire in genetically identical twins correlates with multiple sclerosis. Nature 1993; 364:243-47.

49. Davey MP, Meyer MM, Bakke AC. T-cell receptor Vβ gene expression in monozygotic twins. Discordance in CD8 subset and in disease states. J Immunol 1994; 152:315-21.

50. Dannecker G, Mecheri S, Heuser M et al. Differential expression of T-cell receptor variable β genes on CD4$^+$ and CD8$^+$ T cells: influence by sex linked genes? Immunobiol 1993; 187:17-23.

51. DerSimonian H, Band H, Brenner MB. Increased frequency of T-cell receptor Vα12.1 expression on CD8+ T cells: evidence that Vα participates in shaping the peripheral T-cell repertoire. J Exp Med 1991; 174:639-48.

52. Loveridge JA, Rosenburg WMC, Kirkwood TBL et al. The genetic contribution to human T-cell receptor repertoire. Immunol 1991; 74:246-50.

53. Grunewald J, Janson CH and Wigzell H. Biased expression of individual T-cell receptor V gene segments in CD4$^+$ and CD8$^+$ human peripheral blood T lymphocytes. Eur J Immunol 1991; 21:819-22.

54. Matis LA. The molecular basis of T-cell specificity. Annu Rev Immunol 1990; 8:65-82.

55. Lai E, Concannon P, Hood L. Conserved organization of the human and murine T-cell receptor β-gene families. Nature 1988; 331:543-48.

56. Li V, Szabo P, Posnett DN. The genomic structure of human Vβ6 T-cell antigen receptor genes. J Exp Med 1991; 174:1537-47.

57. Gomolka M, Epplen C, Buitkamp J et al. Novel members and germline polymorphisms in the human T-cell receptor Vβ6 family. Immunogenetics 1993; 37:257-65.

58. Born W, Yagüe J, Palmer E et al. Rearrangement of T-cell receptor β chain genes during T-cell development. Proc Natl Acad Sci 1985; 82:2925-29.

59. Schlissel M, Voronova A, Baltimore D. Helix-loop-helix transcription factor E47 activates immunoglobulin heavy chain germ-line transcription and rearrangement in a pre-T-cell line. Genes Dev 1991; 5:1367-76.

60. Krimpenfort P, De Jong R, Uematsu Y et al. Transcription of T-cell receptor β chain genes is controlled by a downstream regulatory element. EMBO J 1988; 7:745-50.

61. Spolski R, Miescher E, Erard R et al. Regulation and expression of T-cell β chain, L3T4 and Ly-2 messages in Abelson/Molony virus-transformed T-cell lines. Eur J Immunol 1988; 18:295-300.

62. Candeias S, Waltzinger C, Benoist C et al. The Vβ17+ T-cell repertoire: skewed Jβ usage after thymic selection; dissimilar CDR3s in CD4+ versus CD8+ cells. J Exp Med 1991; 174:989-1000.

63. Barth RK, Kim BS, Lan NC, et al. The murine T-cell receptor uses a limited repertoire of expressed Vβ gene segments. Nature 1985; 316:517-23.

64. Hansen T, Qvigstad E, Lundin KEA et al. T-cell receptor β usage by 35 different antigen-specific T-cell clones restricted by HLA-Dw4 or -Dw14.1. Hum Immunol 1992; 35:149-56.

65. Hawes GE, Struyk L, Godthelp BC, Van den Elsen PJ. Limited restriction in the αβTCR V region usage of antigen specific clones: recognition of myelin basic protein (a.a.84-102) and Mycobacterium bovis 65kD heat shock protein (a.a.3-13) by T-cell clones established from PBMC of monozygotic twins and HLA identical individuals. J Immunol 1995; 154:555-66.

66. Van Schooten WCA, Long Ko J, Van der Stoep N et al. T-cell receptor β-chain gene usage in the T-cell recognition of Mycobacterium leprae antigens in one tuberculoid leprosy patient. Proc Natl Acad Sci 1992; 89:11244-248.

67. Struyk L, Kurnick JT, Hawes GE et al. T-cell receptor V-gene usage in synovial fluid lymphocytes of patients with chronic arthritis. Hum Immunol 1993; 37:237-51.

68. Choi Y, Kotzin B, Herron L et al. Interaction of Staphylococcus aureus toxin "superantigens" with human T cell. Proc Natl Acad Sci 1989; 86:8941-45.

69. Oksenberg JR, Stuart S, Begovich AB et al. Limited heterogeneity of rearranged T-cell receptor Vα transcripts in brains of multiple sclerosis patients. Nature 1990; 345:344-46.

70. Wucherpfennig KW, Ota K, Endo N et al. Shared human T-cell receptor Vβ usage to immunodominant regions of myelin basic protein. Science 1990; 248:1016-19.

71. Ferradini L, Roman-Roman S, Azocar J et al. Studies on the human T-cell receptor α/β variable region genes II. Identification of four additional Vβ subfamilies. Eur J Immunol 1991; 21:935-42.

72. Roman-Roman S, Ferradini L, Azocar J et al. Studies on the human T-cell receptor α/β variable region genes. I. Identification of 7 additional Vα subfamilies and 14 Jα segments. Eur J Immunol 1991; 21:927-33.

73. Moore KL. The Developing Human. 1988 Clinically Oriented Embryology, 4th edn. Saunders, Philadelphia.

CHAPTER 3

T CELL RECEPTOR USAGE IN ALLOREACTIVITY

Gail E. Hawes and Peter J. van den Elsen

3. SUMMARY

Under normal circumstances, T cells confer cellular immunity by the specific recognition of peptides of foreign antigens which are presented by self-MHC molecules. The recognition of these peptide/MHC complexes occurs through the clonotypic T cell receptor (TCR). Much attention has been focused on the TCR in the past several years. In particular, the characterization of TCR usage has been of central importance in several T cell mediated autoimmune diseases as well as in the protective immunity against viral and tumor antigens. A significant type of reactivity for which the TCR also has been studied is that of the recognition of allo-MHC molecules, which is relevant for transplantation immunology. Alloreactivity is a very aggressive and prevalent immune response in transplanted allografts and quite often leads to rejection of the graft. Therefore, the analysis of the T cells responsible for this activity could be useful in understanding the nature of alloreactivity in transplantation and might also be useful for the development of specific immune intervention. This review will focus on the TCR usage found in different models of alloreactivity.

3.1 INTRODUCTION

The TCR is composed of a disulfide linked α and β chain that are generated by the recombination of noncontiguous gene segments from pools of variable (V), diversity (D - β only), and joining (J) segments,[1] such that one V(D)J complex is formed. This complex is then juxtaposed to a constant (C) region by RNA splicing. Further variability is added by imprecise joining of the segments and random nucleotide

The Human T-Cell Receptor Repertoire and Transplantation, edited by Peter J. van den Elsen. © 1995 R.G. Landes Company.

addition (N nucleotides).[1-3] Within the α and β chains of the TCR three regions of hypervariability can be discerned. These regions are homologous to the immunoglobulin complementarity determining regions and are likewise designated CDR1, CDR2, and CDR3. Based on this homology and molecular modelling,[4-6] as well as amino acid substitution within these regions,[7] it has been proposed that the CDR1 and CDR2 regions (located within the TCRV gene segments) bind to the α-helices of the MHC molecules while the CDR3 region (the joining between the V(D)J gene segments) recognizes the peptide presented in the context of the MHC on the antigen presenting cell (APC). It was therefore proposed that allo-T cells specific for one particular MHC may share structural similarities.

The T cell response in alloreactivity is quite vigorous in both in vivo responses against allografts as well as in vitro mixed lymphocyte reactions (MLR). It is now commonly accepted that the same pool of T cells responsible for the classical recognition of foreign antigens is also responsible for alloreactivity, rather than independent sets of T cells.[8-10] A relatively high percentage of the T cell compartment (1-10%) is capable of mounting a response to alloantigens.[10-19] The exact mechanisms of allorecognition are still a topic of debate, and there are a number of theories with experimental data to support each one. These range from the direct recognition of the mismatches between host and foreign MHC, to the indirect recognition of peptides of the foreign MHC in the context of self or syngeneic MHC. (reviewed in ref. 8.) It appears likely that a number of different mechanisms are operating simultaneously.

The most frequently discussed mechanism is that of the direct recognition of the foreign MHC alleles being expressed on the allograft. This type of recognition accounts for the majority of the frequent alloreactivity.[15,16] The reactivity toward the mismatched alleles has been thought to be in most cases peptide dependent (if not peptide specific),[19-22] and with the recent delineation of MHC and peptide interactions this is logical in that a particular peptide or set of peptides stabilizes the conformation of the MHC molecule and is expressed as a complex on the cell surface of APC.[23] However it has also been demonstrated that allorecognition of "empty" MHC class I molecules is possible.[24,25] This peptide dependency was initially theorized based on the fact that the fine specificities of certain allo-specific T clones could distinguish between subtypes of MHC alleles which varied at amino acids within the framework of the molecules. More concrete proof of this was shown using peptide inhibition studies. A peptide of influenza virus hemagglutinin which binds to DR1 was able to modulate the allorecognition of some DR1 specific alloclones in a dose-dependent manner.[22] With the delineation of the exact variations within the subtypes of MHC that influence peptide binding, differences in alloreactivity were seen.[26] Later, this was confirmed with more technologically advanced methods where MHC molecules have been altered, such as site directed mutagenesis, in which MHC molecules varied only at amino acids in the β sheet influencing the peptide binding groove. These differing amino acids point toward the peptide bound to the MHC and were therefore not directly available to the TCR for recognition, but rather influence the peptide binding.[27-30] In other studies it has been demonstrated that alterations in the peptide binding site of the MHC alone (thus altering the peptide composition) can reciprocally alter or abrogate alloreactivity.[31,32] This type of reactivity is true for both MHC class I as well as class II molecules.

More recently considered is the reactivity that is more obviously peptide restricted, which is that of indirect allorecognition. This is the recognition of peptides derived from the allogeneic peptide/MHC alleles presented in the context of self or syngeneic MHC. This can take place in the foreign tissue where matching HLA antigens — therefore seen as "self" — can present endogenous peptides from the allograft tissue or from the mismatched HLA antigens as well (allowing acute CTL responses), or can be represented by exogenous peptides of the foreign antigens being taken up by host cells and presented by self APC (resulting in class II restricted responses).[33-39] It has been proposed that this last form of alloreactivity may be the primary cause of chronic rejection,[40] even though the precursor frequency of these alloreactive T cells is much lower than that for direct recognition.[33]

All of these situations exist as in vitro models and the TCR usage has been examined by a number of groups for these various models in hope of defining an effective immunosuppressive strategy for the intervention in allograft rejection to prolong allograft survival. At the very least, defining the TCR repertoire involved in alloreactivity may help to provide answers to the questions that still exist over the precise mechanisms involved.

3.2 TCR ANALYSIS OF GRAFT INFILTRATING T LYMPHOCYTES

Earlier studies focused on the phenotypic and functional analysis of T cells that could be isolated from allograft mononuclear cell infiltrates. T lymphocyte cultures could easily be propagated from renal[41-43] and cardiac[44-47] as well as liver[48] transplant biopsies. A correlation was seen between the amount of T cell infiltrate and rejection.[45,48-50] More importantly, donor specific alloreactivity of MHC class I[41-43,46,47] as well as MHC class II[42-44,46] molecules could be detected in these cultures opening the door to new possibilities of studying the cellular functions of these allospecific T cells in vitro. Using cellular assays, it was postulated that the T cell infiltrates were quite heterogeneous based on the fact that the clones and lines often expressed different fine specificities or cross-reactivities for particular MHC alleles.[29,32]

The specific TCR repertoire analysis of these graft infiltrates became of interest in hope of defining specific characteristics of the repertoire that could be singled out and used for diagnostic as well as therapeutic purposes. By using Southern blot analysis and more recently, polymerase chain reaction (PCR) several groups attempted to define TCR usage and selection in human allograft rejection. Unfortunately, these analyses yielded conflicting results between the different studies. Several reports showed promising results stating that the TCR usage was limited or restricted to "oligoclonal" populations in renal[51-55] as well as cardiac[49,50,55,56] allograft infiltrating T lymphocytes. There appeared to be dominance of a few T cell receptor β chain rearrangements as defined by the Southern blot analysis, but whether this was due to an abundance of T cells from the same progenitor, or from cells sharing a similar T cell receptor β chain rearrangement can not be determined by this type of analysis. The group of Frisman et al.,[55] noted the recurrence of the same TCR rearrangements in sequential biopsies. Miceli et al.,[42,51] also noted a similar recurrence of dominant rearrangements in sequential biopsies and further proposed that in early time points the infiltrate was more limited, then increasing over time becoming more polyclonal. Krams et al.,[57] suggested that this is due to the cytokines produced locally which leads to the recruitment of nonspecific lymphocytes because T cells are responding to multiple epitopes or multiple donor antigens. Other studies, however, found the opposite to be true.[58,59] Even in biopses taken from early time points, the infiltrates were determined to be polyclonal in nature, having many specificities and differing TCRBV region genes. This did not seem to be related to time of biopsy, number of mismatches or the severity of rejection.[59] This is a direct contradiction to the previously mentioned studies. However, one point did remain consistent, which was the correlation between the amount of total mononuclear cell infiltrate within the biopsy to the severity of the rejection episode.

This phenomenon of the same rearrangements occurring in multiple biopsies from different time points was also demonstrated more recently with the more definitive techniques of PCR and DNA sequencing. Hu et al.,[60] have shown that in multiple biopsies the same donor specific TCR clonotypes were present over a period of a few months, even in the absence of an obvious rejection episode. It appeared that the T cells infiltrating the allografted hearts expressed a limited number of TCRBV families, some of which could be traced in T cell lines as well as in peripheral blood samples taken at different time points after transplantation.

3.3. TCR Usage in "Direct" Allorecognition of MHC Molecules

Since studies looking at the lymphocytes infiltrating allografts have shown conflicting results, a more specific examination of the exact clonotypes present in alloreactivity was necessary. Several studies in the past few years have also made use of in vitro mixed lymphocyte reactions (MLRs) to generate T cell lines and clones, representing alloreactivity by direct recognition of foreign MHC alleles, which then could be analyzed by various PCR, and often DNA sequencing, techniques. Therefore, two different lines of approach could be used to delineate alloreactivity: Further analysis of the graft infiltrates by T cell cloning as well as the MLRs were used to generate T cell lines and clones with well defined specificities and cross-reactivities to examine the specific αβTCR repertoire more closely. Tables 3.1 and 3.2 list an overview of these studies. These range from the recognition of MHC class I alleles to a wide variety of MHC class II alleles (mainly DR molecules), as well as subtypes of these alleles, respectively.

3.3.1 TCR usage in the "direct" recognition of MHC class I alleles

As can be seen by the list in Table 3.1, the TCRBV usage in the direct recognition of MHC class I alleles appears to be quite heterogeneous. Individual studies conclude more or less the same findings: The overall patterns were heterogeneous, particularly in the junctional regions, however, the TCRBV usage appears to be non-random or limited. In particular the response against HLA-B27[30,61-63] seems to be predominated by TCRV genes from subgroup 4 as defined by Chothia et al.,[4] particularly TCRBV14, TCRBV13. The amino acid composition of the CDR3 region showed wide diversity, in spite of the conserved TCRV gene segment usage even for T cell clones with the same (overlapping) fine specificities. There was speculation of a conserved alanine residue encoded by N-region nucleotides followed by an acidic amino acid encoded by the TCRBJ gene segment. This could be selectively advantageous for these T cells being specific for a particular set of peptides presented by the B*2705 subtype. A more recent study has also examined the direct recognition of another HLA-B determinant – HLA-B35.[64] In this study, one HLA-B35⁻ responder was used in an MLR. Six T cell clones as well as the original T cell line from which the T cell clones were generated were analyzed for the TCR usage. The T cell clones revealed a different usage of TCRBV and TCRBJ gene segments. However, two of the six clones were found to express highly related sequences with very similar CDR3 regions as well. Another highly similar sequence was found as the dominant population in the T cell line from which the T cell clones were derived. From this the authors concluded that a very restricted TCR usage can dominate an alloresponse.

In the report from Datema et al.[49] it was also concluded that the TCR usage was limited. Six sequential biopsies from a heart allograft were analyzed by PCR for TCRV region usage. Only a few TCRV genes could be amplified out of the biopsies whereas the PBMC from the same patient expressed nearly all of the TCR families. One biopsy taken from a rejection episode also yielded alloreactive T cells specific

Table 3.1. Overview of the current literature regarding direct alloreactivity specific for MHC class I molecules: V gene usage of the TCR

Source	TCR Vβ	N-D-N	Jβ	Vα	Subgroup	Specificity	Usage (Conclusion)	Ref.
16 B27 specific clones from 5 B27⁻ individuals (MLR).	Vβ14	PTTSVR	1.5	?	4	B*2705	Selective Vβ usage. The clones preferentially used a member of subgroup 4. Vα unrestricted completely. The Vβ13's with B*2705 specificity all use Jβ1.1. CDR3's vary overall with a possibly conserved alanine which is followed by an acidic a.a. from Jβ.	30,61-63
	Vβ14	SSQGRLSPGF	1.2	7	4			
	Vβ14	FLAAGVΔ	2.3	1	4			
	Vβ13	PGMAYΔ	1.1	6	4			
	Vβ13	ESRQIΔ	1.1	ND	4			
	Vβ13	RDRTΔ	1.1	15	4			
	Vβ17	IGAIG	2.2	10	4			
	Vβ4	GLAGΔ	2.1	ND	3			
	Vβ4	EQGFVGGΔ	2.5	22	3			
	Vβ15	DLT	2.3	14	4	B*2705 and B*2703		
	Vβ3	KRTQG	2.7	22	4			
	Vβ4	VAGPLI	2.1	1	3	B*2705 and B*2702		
	Vβ4	YSSTGV	2.7	ND	3			
	Vβ5	TRSQ	1.1	7	1			
	Vβ13	YRTGTSA	2.5	ND	4	B*2705, -01		
	Vβ7	HRGGS	2.6	12	2	All but 2703		
1 cardiac transplant patient - 6 sequential bx's.	Vβ6, 7, 8, 14, 17, 18			Vα2, 3, 4, 5, 8, 10, 12, 15, 16, 17, 18			Limited number of V genes used. Cytotoxic activity only found from bx during rejection episode.	49
4 independent sequences derived from clones isolated from bx's.	Vβ	N-D-N	Jβ	Vα	CD4/CD8	HLA-A29	Only one (identical) sequence of clones found that resulted in specific cytotoxicity. Alloreactive clone not found in earlier bx. The rest of the clones were not specifically cytotoxic.	
	Vβ20	VPGA	1.2	Vα10	CD8⁺			
	Vβ6.6/7	LLPL	2.1	Vα5	CD8⁺			
	Vβ14			Vα21	CD4⁺			
	Vβ6.4	LDRP	2.5	Vα4	CD4⁺			
MLR from one B35⁺ responder. 6 T cell clones:	Vβ7.1	EWLGQGIS	2.3	Vα14.1		B35	Restricted usage of TCR α and β based on clones. Two clones use nearly identical α and β chain. Similar, but not identical sequences were also found in the original line.	64
	Vβ4.1	GGVF	2.7	Vα2.3				
	Vβ7.2	ALPLPGMT	2.7	Vα12.1				
	Vβ4.1	GGTI	2.7	Vα2.3				
	Vβ13.2	YQTV	2.3	Vα23.1				
	Vβ22.1	EILQG	1.4	Vα8.1				

for HLA-A29. Cloning of the line and DNA sequencing of the T cell clones revealed that all the clones isolated that were responsible for the specific cytotoxicity were actually identical in sequence and likely from the same progenitor cell. Examination of the material from earlier time points with a probe specific only for the alloreactive clone showed that this clone was not present in the early biopsies. This correlates to the lack of cytotoxic activity in these biopsies and suggests that this clone was recently recruited to the allograft and possibly the direct cause of the rejection episode.

The above mentioned studies have also analyzed the TCRAV usage. It appears that the TCR α chain repertoire was very heterogeneous with absolutely no overlapping TCRAV gene usage apparent related to the allo-response, with the exception of the two nearly identical T cell clones specific for HLA-B35.[64] Similar to the TCRβ chain in this study, this sequence was also predominant in the original T cell line suggesting that this TCRAV together with the TCRBV form the receptor on one T cell clonotype.

3.3.2. TCR usage in the "direct" alloreactivity of MHC class II molecules

MHC class II recognition in alloreactivity has been more extensively studied. Table 3.2 gives an overview of the current findings regarding the TCRV region usage in this response. Several of these studies have not been concerned with the different MHC class II molecules but rather have looked at the variation in the recognition of the different subtypes within particular molecules. Mostly these studies are using MLRs between mismatched responder/stimulator combinations where the responder does not carry a subtype of the HLA class II haplotype in question. However, a few studies also included responder/stimulator pairs with subtypes from the same HLA class II molecule to determine if there is a difference in the allo-response when the responder also expresses an HLA class II haplotype closely related or nearly identical to the donor. The most extensively studied are HLA-DR1 and DR4, and to a lesser extent DR2, DR5, DQ8 and DP2.

Four independent studies are listed that have studied the T cell reactivity against DR1. Hand et al.,[65] have examined the TCRBV gene usage in a biopsy from a renal allograft where the T cells were specific for the DR1 alloantigen. The analysis suggested a specific outgrowth of primarily TCRBV8 followed by TCRBV5S1, and TCRBV4. To test this result, the experiment was followed up by two trials of MLR from the same responder/donor combination. The predominant usage of TCRBV8 was found in both reactions thus strengthening the suggestion of a selective advantage of TCRBV8 in the allorecognition of DR1. From this it was postulated that MLR could be a useful tool in predicting the specific response of alloreactivity in transplantation. Other studies have examined the TCRV gene usage in the DR1 response in

Table 3.2. Overview of the current literature regarding direct alloreactivity specific for MHC class II molecules: V gene usage of the TCR

Population analyzed:	TCR usage:					Specificity	Usage (Conclusion)[b]	Ref.
	Vβ	N-D-N	Jβ	Vα	Subgroup[a]			
2 DR1- donors used to generate clones.	Vβ5.1	SFMTPG	1.1	17.1	1	DR1	Heterogeneous usage with some overlapping in V genes. The overall N-D-N is highly variable. No correlation between TCR gene usage and DR1 alloreactivity was identified.	66
	Vβ18.1	SPGPDLNS	2.2	21.1	1			
	Vβ5.1	SSWTGLG	1.2	21.1	1			
	Vβ4.2	ESILAK	2.1	?	3			
	Vβ4.1	EGGMGD	2.7	8.2	3			
	Vβ2.1	PQGGT	1.2	ND	3			
	Vβ3.3	SLSRTS	1.4	14.1	4			
	Vβ3.1	---	1.6	10.1	4			
6 individual responders, 11 clones. S14 (DR1):	Vβ2.1	SKTGRG	2.7	17.1	(3)	DRB1*0101	Diverse but non-random usage of V genes. There is some overlap between individuals. J genes as well as N-D-N regions are very diverse.	28
	Vβ2.1	ASTAS	2.1	2.6	(3)			
	Vβ4.1	VAGQGTD	2.7	?	(3)			
	Vβ18.1	PTV	2.7	22.1	(1)			
	Vβ5.1	STTSGSN	2.7	8.1	(1)	DRB1*0101 & 0102		
AL61 (DR1):	Vβ5.1	KEPRG	1.5	17.1	(1)	DRB1*0101		
	Vβ5.5	LMGDRG	1.6	22.1	(1)			
AL62 (DR1):	Vβ5-like	LGQGT	2.7	13.1	(1)	DRB1*0101		
S26 (DR1+):	Vβ4.1	VEDRDRV	2.1	13.1	(3)	DRB1*0101		
S30 (DR1+):	Vβ17.1	SLDSW	2.3	19.1	(4)	DRB1*0101		
S25 (DR1+):	Vβ2.1	LGTGS	1.2	13.1	(3)	DRB1*0102		
7 clones from 3 DR1- responders. N:	Vβ6.7c	RNRRLLAD	2.3	ND		DRB1*0103	Based on these clones, it is predictable that analysis of alloreactivity will show preferential V gene segment usage associated with the involvement of different CDR regions in the contact with a defined MHC epitope.	67
	Vβ6.7a	WGWA	2.4	ND				
P:	Vβ8.3b	SQTP	1.1	ND		*0103 & DRw13		
A/G:	Vβ8.3a	GQG	1.5	ND		*0103,w13,DR4w10		
	Vβ13	NG	1.1	ND		DRw13,DR4w10		
	Vβ13.2	EGGW	1.1	ND		DRw13,DR4w10		
	Vβ13	EAMAG	1.2	ND		DRw13		
Renal bx, donor specific T cell line. Primary MLR conducted twice with donor/recipient pair to confirm.	Bx PCR: **Vβ8, Vβ5.1, Vβ4** 1° MLR: **Vβ8, Vβ6** 1° MLR: **Vβ8, Vβ3**					DR1	Selective advantage of Vβ8. MLR also gave Vβ8, demonstrating predictive potential of MLR and PCR.	65

Population analyzed:	TCR usage:					Specificity	Usage (Conclusion)[b]	Ref.
	Vβ	N-D-N	Jβ	Vα	Subgroup[a]			
1 responder (DR3 Dw3,DR4 Dw4) used for 1 line and 2 clones.	Vβ8.2 Vβ8.2	SQGPT TSGT	2.2 2.3	ND ND		DR4 Dw14	Vβ8 was dominant in the line, and both clones were also Vβ8. The CDR3's were very diverse.	68
12 responders (DR4 + and -) were used to generate lines and clones against DR4 subtypes. 102 clones αDRB1*0404 from *0401+ 60 clones α-*0404 from *0401- 26 clones α-*0403 from *0401+	Vβ usage of clones αDRB1*0404 (from DRB1*0401+) **Vβ6** 26% Vβ13.2 10% Vβ2 10% Vβ18 9% Vβ5.2 9%	8 of 9 individuals 4 of 9 individuals 6 of 9 individuals 3 of 9 individuals 3 of 9 individuals		ND ND		DRB1*0404 (DR4Dw14.1)	Preferential usage of Vβ6 in both DR4+ and DR4- individuals. The second most used Vβ was more individual specific.	69, 70
	Vβ usage of clones αDRB1*0404 (from DRB1*0401-) **Vβ6** 8% Vβ2 6.5% Vβ18 4% Vβ13.2 3%		Vβ5.2 3% Vβ5.1 3% Vβ7 3%			DRB1*0404 (DR4Dw14.1)		
	Vβ usage of clones αDRB1*0403 (from DRB1*0401+) Vβ4 27% Vβ13.1 19% Vβ20 15%		Vβ5.1 12% Vβ13.2 8% Vβ6 2%			DRB1*0403 (DR4Dw13.1)		
Vβ6+ clones were chosen for sequencing from 3 responders:	**Vβ**	**N-D-N**	**Jβ**	**Vα**				
BAJ (DR4+)	Vβ6.1 Vβ6.6/7 Vβ6.6/7 Vβ6.8/9	RLTDQGGSP LGTEGGR LTTGGG E	2.5 2.7 2.7 1.1	ND ND ND ND				
FAR (DR4+)	Vβ6.6/7 Vβ6.6/7 Vβ6.8/9 Vβ6.8/9 Vβ6.?	LSS TGRTGRD LLFQG LTLQG RLA5VGVPR	2.1 1.2 1.1 1.1 2.5	ND ND ND ND ND				
LAB (DR4-)	Vβ6.2/3 Vβ6.6/7 Vβ6.6/7 Vβ6.6/7	TFGG QY Q RTD	1.5 2.7 2.1 1.2	ND ND ND ND				

(continued)

(Table 3.2. continued)

Population analyzed:	TCR usage:					Specificity	Usage (Conclusion)[b]	Ref.
	Vβ	N-D-N	Jβ	Vα	Subgroup[a]			
Vβ8+ cells were sorted from a DR1+ responder. 4 clones were generated	Vβ8.2 Vβ8.1	LATGLIY LGAALLK	2.7 1.2	ND ND		DR5	Vβ8 clones suggested that allo-reactivity is quite diverse.	71
	Vβ8.2 Vβ8.2	PKSRYTL LLYRQGN	1.1 1.6	ND ND		DR2		
2 identical clones with dual alloreactivity DR2/B27 specific.	Vβ1.1	PRTGL	1.1	ND		DR2	B27 activity is CD8/cl.I restricted DR2 activity is cl.II restricted.	63
4 clones derived from a DQw7+ responder.	Vβ7.1 Vβ5.1 Vβ8.2 Vβ5.3	QVAGLEYP LTSRPWY SGGY LVTGRA	2.3 2.5 2.3 2.3	2.1/4.1a 3.1 21.1a 20.1		DQw8	Possible preferential usage of certain TCR structures - CDR1 motif, conserved Jβ. All used different Vα and β's.	73
Tertiary MLR: responder/stimulator differ only at the DP locus.	3 of 9 clones used **Vβ14**, the other 6 clones used all different Vβ's based on southern blots.					DPw2	Increased usage of Vβ14, however 2nd individual showed no Vβ14. (Data not shown.)	72

a. The subgroup is based on the criteria outlined in Chothia, et.al.[4] The subgroups listed in parentheses have not been discussed in the reference but have been included in the table by the authors of this review for comparison purposes.

b. The conclusions listed in this column are a summarization of the conclusions drawn by the authors of the particular articles referenced and may vary from the conclusions in this review as discussed in the text.

more detail by the DNA sequencing of T cell clones.[28,66,67] Geiger et al.,[66] used two responders that did not express the DR1 haplotype to generate clones against DR1 molecules. They concluded that the overall response was heterogeneous in TCRV gene usage as well as in the CDR3 regions of these clones. They also did not observe any usage of TCRBV8 as in the study of Hand et al.[65] The two other studies were even more detailed in examining the fine specificities of clones which could distinguish between subtypes of DR1. Champagne et al.,[67] also concluded that MLR could be useful as a prediction of preferential usage of TCRV gene segments in association with the involvement of different CDR regions in the contact with a defined MHC epitope. This was based on T cell clones isolated from three DR1⁻ individuals with varying overlaps in specificity. Two T cell clones which were specific for DRB1*0103 only, used the TCRBV6 gene segment. Two T cell clones that recognized both DRB1*0103 and DRw13 (one also recognized DR4Dw10) used the TCRBV8 gene segment — which interestingly was the preferentially used TCRBV gene segment in the study by Hand et al.[65] The last three T cell clones were specific for DRw13 — two of which reacted with Dw18 and Dw19 as well as cross-reacted with DR4Dw10 also, whereas the other clone reacted only with Dw19. All three of these T cell clones used the TCRBV13 gene segment. The CDR3 regions of these clones were all very diverse even when clones shared TCRBV usage and MHC specificity. It appeared that the TCRBV usage was conserved in clones with overlapping specificity, however the number of T cell clones is very limited and furthermore the T cell clones with the same fine specificity were derived from one individual. Therefore, an individual specific preferential response cannot be excluded on the basis of this study. Katovich-Hurley et al.,[28] have also looked at DR1 alloresponses in a similar manner. Eleven clones were generated from six individuals, of which, three were DR1⁻ and three were DR1⁺. This was termed broad and narrow priming, respectively. They concluded that the response in these individuals was diverse but non-random in that there was some overlap in TCRBV gene usage. TCRBV2, 4, and 5 were the most frequently used, which corresponds to the study of Geiger, et al.,[66] where TCRBV2, 4, or 5 are used by five of the eight clones. The significance of this is debatable, as these TCRBV genes are from different subgroups according to the classification by Chothia et al.[4] (TCRBV5 is subgroup 1, TCRBV2 and TCRBV4 are subgroup 3) and therefore have less structural homology with each other. Furthermore, these TCRV genes are also normally quite abundant in the periphery of most individuals, thus maybe having a selective advantage purely through sheer numbers.

The CDR3 regions in the TCR were overall very diverse once again, however they did find two T cell clones with shared amino acid usage in the N-Dβ-N region and identical TCRAV usage. These two clones used different TCRBV genes and also exhibited different fine specificities.

It is possible that the peptide being recognized is similar for these clones and the difference in the TCRBV usage corresponds to the differences in fine specificities in the HLA recognition as the authors discussed. There also appeared to be no difference in the overall TCR usage when comparing the broad and narrow priming condition. However, the number of T cell clones that could be generated from the narrow priming is much smaller when compared to the broad priming condition.[28] This could be related to the effects of selection processes which occur in the thymus that shape the available circulating T cell repertoire. One would expect the cross-reactivity between fine specificities to be greater between the subtypes of one particular DR haplotype. Therefore in the DR1+ individuals (narrow priming) the bulk of potential alloreactive clones would cross-react with self MHC molecules and be eliminated during thymic maturation, resulting in a smaller population of T cells available that are capable of responding to allo-antigen of a similar subtype as the responder. Overall, it appears that the response to DR1 alloantigens is largely a diverse set of T cells with preferential usage of TCRBV genes belonging to subgroups 1 and 3.

DR4 allorecognition has also been analyzed for TCR usage. The first of these studies used a DR4Dw4 responder to examine the response against DR4Dw14, also a narrow priming experiment. Similar to Hand et al.[65] for the DR1 recognition, Yamanaki et al.,[68] also found a dominant usage of TCRBV8 against DR4Dw14. The specific line was analyzed by PCR and clearly the TCRBV8 family was the predominant TCRBV while others were present but greatly diminished. Two T cell clones with the same specificity as the original T cell line were both TCRBV8S2 confirming the PCR analysis from the T cell line. From this we can already conclude that a particular TCRBV predominance is not uniquely associated with a specific MHC molecule, as both DR1 and DR4 subtypes can select for TCRBV8.

The TCRBV8 is not found back in the extensive panel of DR4 alloreactive clones from Goronzy et al.[69,70] This panel was also concerned with the activity against DR4Dw14 (DRB1*0404). The response against DRB1*0404 was compared between DRB1*0401+ and DRB1*0401- individuals as well as to the response of DRB1*0401+ individuals against a different subtype of DR4 - DRB1*0403. A total of 162 T cell clones from 12 responders specific for DRB1*0404 were examined for TCRBV usage. A clear trend was seen in both DR4+ and DR4- responders. TCRBV6 dominated the response in both groups when all T cell clones were regarded together as a whole, although the percentages of TCRBV6 usage were different between the two groups (26% for DR4+ responders compared to 8% in DR4- responders). The overall relative pattern of most frequent to least frequent TCRBV genes used was nearly identical between these groups. On an individual basis, TCRBV6 was the most dominant TCRBV gene in nearly all responders, however, the second most dominant TCRBV gene varied between responders and was largely individual specific. The TCRBV gene usage against the DRB1*0403 subtype was clearly different with TCRBV4 dominating and only a very low amount of TCRBV6 present (2%). It is interesting to note that no significant amounts of the TCRBV8 were seen as in the other studies as might have been expected. To examine the preferential usage of TCRBV6 in more detail, a number of TCRBV6[+] clones were sequenced. The specific TCRBV and TCRBJ genes used as well as the amino acid usage of the CDR3 regions demonstrated great diversity in the junctional regions even within this restricted group of T cell clones.

The studies examining the response against other MHC class II molecules is rather limited. Wilson et al.,[71] have taken a different approach and started with a particular TCRBV gene — TCRBV8 — from a DR1[+] individual and tested for alloreactivity against the different DR molecules. Based on the other studies discussed here, one might expect that DR1 and DR4 stimulators would elicit a response, however, in this panel, that was not the case. The initial TCRBV8 T cell line was tested for primary alloreactivity before specific selection. A low level of activity was present against DR3 only. Then the T cell lines were selectively activated with DR2 or DR5 homozygous B cell lines. A very efficient and non-overlapping or cross-reacting response was generated against the respective DR molecules demonstrating that generating allospecific T cell lines from a very specific subset of the T cell compartment is possible. T cell clones from these T cell lines revealed once again diversity in the junctional regions of the TCR expressed by allospecific T cells.

Reports over the T cell response against DP and DQ molecules in regards to TCR usage have reached conclusions similar to the those drawn from the DR studies. It was shown that there was a possible preferential usage of a particular TCRBV gene (TCRBV14 - DPw2).[72] Also TCRBV genes with similarities in the CDR1 region (DQw8) with diversity in the junctional regions were found.[73]

3.4. TCR USAGE IN "INDIRECT" ALLOREACTIVITY

Fewer studies have been conducted regarding the indirect recognition of peptides of allogeneic MHC molecules than compared to direct recognition. Table 3.3. lists an overview of the results. These studies regard the specific recognition of DRB1*0101 a.a. 21-42, in the context of DRB1*1101.[33,74] A more restricted TCRBV usage is apparent when compared to direct alloreactivity. This is represented in at least four different responders with different sources of stimulators. There was a consensus that TCRBV13S2 preferentially responded to this peptide/MHC combination. Each individual also had other TCRBVs expressed in the T cell lines. These TCRBV genes also occurred preferentially in that there was a shared usage by T cell clones from different individuals: TCRBV13S1 (n=3), TCRBV3 (n=2), TCRBV1 (n=2). Furthermore, one individual also used TCRBV7 (albeit to a lesser extent) which was preferentially used in another individual in response to the DRB1*0101 a.a. 21-42.[75] However this was in the context of DRB1*0101, which is actually a "self" response. So it appears that the less frequent indirect recognition of alloantigens is accomplished by a restricted set of TCRs which is dependent on the presenting molecule, however the number of T cell clones examined to date remains small, and these are specific for one particular peptide/MHC combination. It would also be interesting to know the composition of the CDR3 regions of the T cells responsible for this recognition to determine if only the TCRBV gene is selected or if also particular amino acids in the N-D-N regions are selected biased toward the particular peptide in question, and furthermore, would these CDR3s change if other peptides were presented by the DRB1*1101 in a similar study. Finally, it also remains to be seen if this holds true for other alleles or subtypes of alleles.

3.5. Discussion

Alloreactivity still remains to be a very dominant and life threatening response in allograft recipients. Overall immune suppression has been the general route for treatment, but the treatment itself can also lead to problems and be directly or indirectly fatal. Therefore the need to develop safer, less toxic, more specific therapies are still present. Animal models for T cell mediated diseases spawned a new generation of research focusing on the specific immune receptors responsible for causing disease. The EAE model had offered very promising results where it was shown that the disease initiation was carried out by a very small, restricted set of T cells all expressing a common component — the TCRBV gene — in the T cell receptor (TCR).[76-78] Specific

Table 3.3. Overview of the current literature regarding indirect alloreactivity: V gene usage of the TCR

Source	Vβ	Vα	Usage	Specificity	Restriction	
Peptide stimulation with DR1a.a.21-42. 1 responder: Line and 2 clones	LS:Vb**13.2**, Vb12-weak	ND	Limited usage (PCR only). Both clones Vb13.2.	DRB1*0101 a.a.21-42	DRB1*1101	
3 DRB1*1101[+] responders: peptide stimulation with DR1a.a.21-42	RR:**13.2**, 13.1, 7, 3 BH:**13.2**, 3, 13.1, 1 PR:**13.2**, (13.1)	ND	Limited usage: 3 Individuals—all used Vb13.2 predominantly (PCR only).	DRB1*0101 a.a.21-42	DRB1*1101	
Clones specific for DR1a.a.21-42, presented by DR1.	7 clones: Vb7 2 clones:Vb19 - DR1 restricted but not peptide 21-42 specific.	ND	Restricted. No sequence data, therefore postulated that clones may be from the same progenator cell.	DRB1*0101 a.a.21-42	DRB1*0101	

treatments based on blocking T cells with this particular TCRV gene such as monoclonal antibody or anti-idiotype immune cells were successful at ameliorating the disease process. Furthermore, naive animals could be protected against disease development by vaccination. This was very exciting for T cell immunologists, and the quest for similar specific agents in human diseases began, including transplantation immunology. Attempts have been made at the specific immune regulation or modulation of alloreactive T cells such as monoclonal antibodies directed at various T cell surface structures, soluble immune receptors and natural receptor antagonists (reviewed in ref. 79.).

After reviewing the collection of data regarding the TCR usage in various models of alloreactivity, it becomes clear that the initial postulation that very defined specific oligoclonal subsets of T cells were responsible for alloreactivity is not so simple as in the earlier animal models for T cell mediated diseases. In general, most of the studies conclude that the T cell receptor repertoire is limited or restricted either in the amount of different TCRV genes that are used or in the TCR subgroups used, within which the TCRV genes have a high degree of structural similarities with each other, particularly in the CDR1 and CDR2 regions. However, this restricted TCR usage generally does not seem to be consistent between studies for the same MHC molecule. Furthermore, there seems to be considerable variation between individuals. Granted, it is difficult to make comparisons between such studies because often different T cell culture methods have been used and differences in the time of sampling and patient characteristics other than HLA typing are not taken into consideration. Even so, it appears that if specific anti-T cell therapies were to be developed based on specific TCRV genes, it is reasonable to say that patients would have to be assessed on an individual basis to determine that individual's particular pattern of immune response. This seems to be true of many other studies on human T cell mediated diseases, particularly autoimmune diseases such as RA (reviewed in ref. 80), which is disappointing compared to the early animal models.

It is also not known if specific anti-T cell therapy would be effective with long-term results within alloreactivity. It is quite possible that when the predominant TCRV gene is immunosuppressed, another will take over the response. The results shown for the allorecognition of MHC class I epitopes may offer a more realistic target for direct immunosuppression against particular T cells as compared to MHC class II allorecognition in that the class I alloresponses were fairly restricted regarding TCR usage — more so than the class II alloresponse. This could be a general phenomenon of class I responses resulting from the strict peptide binding properties of class I MHC molecules. It has been shown in other models such as the response against the influenza virus, that the response against MHC class I restricted peptides yields a very limited TCR repertoire which is fairly consistent between individuals.[81-83] However, to correlate this to the restricted response in alloreactivity, one would have to assume that only a very limited set of peptides could be recognized in alloreactivity. A wider set of specifically recognized peptides would be expected to yield a broader range in the TCR that are capable of responding. Although, if the peptide functions more as a stabilizer for the conformation of the MHC molecule rather being specifically recognized, then more variation could be introduced into the peptide pool, still giving rise to a restricted TCR repertoire responding.

Based on the results from the studies reviewed here, it appears that the alloresponse to MHC class II determinants is more heterogenous than that against class I molecules. Again this fits with the current trends being shown in various models for studying TCR response to peptide/MHC complexes. We have shown in our own laboratory that by stimulating PBMC from unprimed individuals with a single MHC class II presented peptide, several different TCRs with differing TCRV genes are capable of responding, with very little overlap in TCRV gene usage between individuals.[84] This panel of control individuals made use of pairs of monozygotic twins as well as HLA identical siblings to examine the effects of the expression and identity of MHC and non-MHC factors on the responding TCR repertoire. Even within a set of twins, a large variation was seen in the response to a single peptide. In an allograft, multiple potential immunoreactive epitopes are present, thus it seems likely that a wide range of T cells would also be present that could mount a response against any or all of these epitopes.

Other approaches to interrupting the T cell activation and homing pathways may lead to more effective, general therapies, eliminating the need to specifically tailor treatments to every patient. More understanding of the early inflammatory processes and events leading to CTL induction such as lymphocyte chemotaxis and adhesion, as well as antigen processing and presentation may offer better results. For instance, examining cytokine profiles and patterns within allografts and for the different types of rejection may lead to effective targeting of these molecules for immunotherapy.[85] One exciting new field of research that is now being examined for use as an immunosuppressive agent in allograft rejection as well as other inflammatory processes, is that of antisense oligonucleotides. Stepkowski et al.,[86] have nicely demonstrated the potential use for blocking adhesion molecules by antisense-oligos. They found that mouse ICAM-1 antisense oligonucleotides inhibited the rejection of heterotropic cardiac allografts. This could also function synergistically with more traditional immunosuppressive drugs currently being used in transplantation, with the exception of cyclosporin A. Furthermore, when using this in combination with monoclonal antibodies against another adhesion molecule — LFA-1, they were able to induce donor specific transplantation tolerance. They conclude that antisense technology offers a new non-toxic, specific immunosuppressive treatment for organ transplantation. It will be interesting to see how this technology's effectiveness develops as it is adapted to the human system.

REFERENCES

1. Hunkapiller T and Hood L. Diversity of the immunoglobulin gene superfamily. Adv Immunol 1989; 44:1-63.
2. Toyanaga B, Yoshikai Y, Vadasz V, et al. Organization and sequences of the diversity, joining, and constant region genes of the human T cell receptor β chain. Proc Natl Acad Sci USA 1985; 82:8624-28.
3. Wilson RK, Lai E, Concannon P, et al. Structure, organization, and polymorphism of murine and human T cell receptor α and β chain gene families. Immunol Rev 1988; 101:149-72.
4. Chothia C, Boswell DR, and Lesk AM. The outline structure of the T-cell αβ receptor. EMBO 1988; 7:3745-55.
5. Claverie J-M, Prochnicka-Chalufour A, and Bougueleret L. Implications of Fab-like structure for the T cell receptor. Immunol Today 1989; 10:10-4.
6. Prochnicka-Chalufour A, Casanova J-I, Avrameas S, et al. Biased amino acid distributions in regions of the T cell receptors and MHC molecules potentially involved in their association. Int Immunol 1991; 3:853-64.
7. Jorgensen JL, Esser U, Fazekas de St. Groth B, et al Mapping T cell receptor-peptide contacts by variant peptide immunization of single-chain transgenics. Nature 1992; 355:224-30.
8. Sherman LA and Chattopadhyay S. The molecular basis of allorecognition. Annu Rev Immunol 1993; 11:385-402.
9. Matis LA, Sorger SB, McElligott DL, et al. The molecular basis of alloreactivity in antigen-specific major histocompatibility complex-restricted T cell clones. Cell 1987; 51:59-69.
10. Lechler RI, Lombardi G, Batchelor JR, et al. The molecular basis of alloreactivity. Immmunol. Today 1990; 11:83-8.
11. Fischer-Lindahl K and Wilson DB. Histocompatibility antigen-activated cytotoxic T lymphocytes. II. Estimates of the frequency and specificity of precursors. J Exp Med 1977; 145:503.
12. Matzinger P and Bevan MJ. Hypothesis: why do so many lymphocytes respond to major histocompatibility antigens. Cell Immunol 1977; 29:1-5.
13. Wilson DB, Bluthe JL, and Nowell PC. Quantitative studies on the mixed lymphocyte reaction: III. Kinetics of the response. J Exp Med 1968 128:1157.
14. Bishop DK and Orosz CG. Limiting dilution analysis for alloreactive, TCGF-secretory T cells. Transplantation 1989; 47:671-7.
15. Sharrock CEM, Man S, Wanachiwanawin W, et al. Analysis of the alloreactive T cell repertoire in man. Transplantation 1987; 43:699-703.
16. Kaminski E, Sharrock C, Hows J, et al. Frequency analysis of cytotoxic T lymphocyte precursors — possible relevance to HLA-matched unrelated donor bone marrow transplantation. Bone Marrow Transplant 1988; 3:149-55.

17. Deacock SJ, Schwarer AP, Bridge J, et al. Evidence that umbilical cord blood contains a higher frequency of HLA class II - specific alloreactive T cells than adult peripheral blood. Transplantation 1992; 53:1128-34.

18. Ashwell JD, Chen C, and Schwartz RH. High frequency and nonrandom distribution of alloreactivity in T cell clones selected for recognition of foreign antigen in association with self class II molecules. J Immunol 1986; 136:389-95.

19. Lombardi G, Sidhu S, Batchelor JR, et al. Allorecognition of DR1 by T cells from a DR4/Dw13 responder mimics self-restricted recognition of endogenous peptides. Proc Natl Acad Sci USA 1989; 86:4190-4.

20. Demotz S, Sette A, Sakaguchi K, et al. Self peptide requirement for class II major histocompatibility complex allorecognition. Proc Natl Acad Sci USA 1991; 88:8730-4.

21. Rojo S, Lopez D, Calvo V, et al. Conservation and alteration of HLA-B27-specific T cell epitopes on mouse cells: implications for peptide-mediated alloreactivity. J Immunol 1991 146:634-42.

22. Eckels DD, Gorski J, Rothbard J, et al. Peptide-mediated modulation of T-cell allorecognition. Proc Natl Acad Sci USA 1988; 85:8191-5.

23. Rötzschke O, Falk K, Faath S, et al. On the nature of peptides involved in T cell alloreactivity. J Exp Med 1991; 174:1059-71.

24. Elliott TJ and Eisen HN. Cytotoxic T lymphocytes recognize a reconstituted class I histocompatibility antigen (HLA-A2) as an allogeneic target molecule. Proc Natl Acad Sci USA 1990; 87:5213-7.

25. Müllbacher A, Hill AB, Blanden RV, et al. Alloreactive cytotoxic T cells recognize MHC class I antigen without peptide specificity. J Immunol 1991 147:1765-72.

26. Demotz S, Barbey C, Corradin G, et al. The set of naturally processed peptides displayed by DR molecules is tuned by polymorphism of residue 86. Eur J Immunol 1993; 23:425-32.

27. Coppin HL, Carmichael P, Lombardi G, et al. Position 71 in the α helix of the DRβ domain is predicted to influence peptide binding and plays a central role in allorecognition. Eur J Immunol 1993; 23:343-9.

28. Katovich-Hurley C, Steiner N, Wagner A, et al. Nonrandom T cell receptor usage in the allorecognition of HLA-DR1 microvariation. J Immunol 1993; 150:1314-24.

29. Santamaria P, Boyce-Jacino MT, Lindstrom AL, et al. Alloreactive T cells can distinguish between the same human class II MHC products on different B cell lines. J Immunol 1991; 146:1822-8.

30. Lopez de Castro JA, Bragado R, Lauzurica P, et al. Structure and immue recognition of HLA-B27 antigens: implications for disease association. Scand J Rheumatol 1990; Suppl.87:21-31.

31. Villadangos JA, Galocha B, and Lopez de Castro JA. Unusual topology of an HLA-B27 allospecific T cell epitope lacking peptide specificity. J Immunol 1994; 152:2317-23.

32. Rosen-Bronson S, Yu W-Y, and Karr RW. Polymorphic HLA-DR7β1 chain residues that are involved in T cell allorecognition. J Immunol 1991; 146:4264-70.

33. Liu Z, Braunstein NS, and Suciu-Foca N. Cell recognition of allopeptides in context of syngeneic MHC. J Immunol 1992; 148:35-40.

34. Fangmann J, Dalchau R, and Fabre JW. Recognition of skin allografts by indirect allorecognition of donor class I major histocompatibility complex peptides. J Exp Med 1992; 175:1521-9.

35. Benichou G, Takizawa PA, Olson CA, et al. Donor major histocompatibility complex (MHC) peptides are presented by recipient MHC molecules during graft rejection. J Exp Med 1992; 175:305-8.

36. Kourilsky P, Chaouar G, Rabourdin-Combe C, et al. Working principles in the immune system implied by the "peptide self" model. Proc Natl Acad Sci USA 1987; 84:3400-4.

37. Pierres M, Marchetto S, Naquet PM, et al. I-A α polymorphic residues that determine alloreactive T cell recognition. J Exp Med 1989; 169:1655-68.

38. De Koster HS, Anderson DC, and Termijtelen A. T cells sensitized to synthetic HLA-DR3 peptide give evidence of continuous presentation of denatured HLA-DR3 molecules by HLA-DP. J Exp Med 1989; 169:1191-6.

39. De Koster HS, van Rood JJ, and Termijtelen A. HLA-DR peptide-induced alloreactive T cell lines reveal an HLA-DR sequence that can be both "dominant" and "cryptic": evidence for allele-specific processing. Eur J Immunol 1992; 22:1531-9.

40. Bradley JA, Mowat MM, and Bolton EM. Processed MHC class I alloantigen as the stimulus for CD4⁺ T-cell dependent antibody-mediated graft rejection. Immunol Today 1992; 13:434-8.

41. Mayer TG, Fuller AA, Fuller TC, et al. Characterization of in vivo-activated allospecific T lymphocytes propagated from human renal allograft biopsies undergoing rejection. J Immunol 1985; 134:258-64.

42. Miceli MC, Barry TS, and Finn OJ. Human allograft-derived T-cell lines: Donor class I- and class II- directed cytotoxicity and repertoire stability in sequential biopses. Human Immunol 1988; 22:185-98.

43. Vandekerckhove BAE, Datema G, Koning F, et al. Analysis of the donor-specific cytotoxic T lymphocyte repertoire in a patient with a long term surviving allograft. J Immunol 1990; 144:1288-94.

44. Zeevi A, Fung J, Zerbe TR, et al. Allospecificity of activated T cells grown from endomyocardial biopsies from heart transplant patients. Transplantation 1986; 41:620-6.

45. Kaufman CL, Zeevi A, Kormos RL, et al. Propagation of infiltrating lymphocytes and graft coronary disease in cardiac transplant recipients. Human Immunol 1990; 28:228-36.

46. Ouwehand AJ, Vaessen LMB, Baan CC, et al. Alloreactive lymphoid infiltrates in human heart transplants: Loss of class II-directed cytotoxicity more than 3 months after transplantation. Human Immunol 1991; 30:50-9.

47. Trentin L, Zambello R, Faggian G, et al. Phenotypic and functional characterization of cytotoxic cells derived from endomyocardial biopsies in human cardiac allografts. Cell Immunol 1992; 141:332-41.
48. Saidman SL, Demetris AJ, Zeevi A, et al. Propagation of lymphocytes infiltrating human liver allografts. Transplantation 1990; 49:107-11.
49. Datema G, Vaessen LMB, Daane RC, et al. Functional and molecular characterization of graft-infiltrating T lymphocytes propagated from different biopsies derived from one heart transplant patient. Transplantation 1994; 57:1119-26.
50. Wyngaard PLJ, Tuynman WB, Gmelig Meyling FH, et al. Endomyocardial biosies after heart transplantation. Transplantation 1993; 55:103-10.
51. Miceli MC and Finn OJ. T cell receptor β-chain selection in human allograft rejection. J Immunol 1989; 142:81-6.
52. Miceli MC, Barry TS, and Finn OJ. Human renal allograft infiltrating T cells: Phenotype-function correlation and clonal heterogeneity. Transplantation Proc 1988; 20:199-201.
53. Hand SL, Hall BL, and Finn OJ. T cell receptor gene usage and expression in renal allograft-derived T cell lines. Human Immunol 1990; 28:82-95.
54. Hall BL and Finn OJ. T cell receptor Vβ gene usage in allograft-derived cell lines analyzed by a polymerase chain reaction technique. Transplantation 1992; 53:1088-99.
55. Frisman DM, Hurwitz AA, Bennett WT, et al. Clonal analysis of graft-infiltrating lymphocytes from renal and cardiac biopses: Dominant rearrangements of TCRβ genes and persistence of dominant rearrangements in serial biopses. Human Immunol 1990; 28:208-15.
56. Datema G, Vaessen LMB, Daane CR, et al. T-cell receptor V gene segment usage of graft-infiltrating T-lymphocytes after heart transplantation. Transplantation Proc 1993; 25:77-9.
57. Krams SM, Falco DA, Villanueva JC, et al. Cytokine and T cell receptor gene expression at the site of allograft rejection. Transplantation 1992; 53:151-6.
58. Bonneville M, Moisan JP, Moreau JF, et al. TRG alpha, beta, and gamma gene rearrangements in human alloreactive T cell clones extracted from a rejected kidney. Transplantation Proc 1988; 20:196-8.
59. Yard BA, Kooymans-Couthino M, Reterink T, et al. Analysis of T cell lines from rejecting renal allografts. Kidney Int 1993; 43(suppl.39):S133-8.
60. Hu H, de Jonge N, Doornewaard H, et al. Cytotoxic T lymphocytes infiltrating the human cardiac allograft show a restriction in T-cell receptor Vβ gene usage: A study on serial biopsy and blood specimens. J Heart Lung Transplant 1994; 13:1058-71.
61. Bragado R, Lauzurica P, Lopez D, et al. T cell receptor Vβ gene usage in human alloreactive response. J Exp Med 1990; 171:1189-1204.
62. Lauzurica P, Bragado R, Lopez D, et al. Asymmetric selection of T cell antigen receptor α-and β-chains in HLA-B27 alloreactivity. J Immunol 1992; 148:3624-30.

63. Lopez D, Barber DF, Villadangos JA, et al. Cross-reactive T cell clones from unrelated individuals reveal similarities in peptide presentation between HLA-B27 and HLA-DR2. J Immunol 1993; 150:2675-86.

64. Steinle A, Reinhardt C, Jantzer P, et al. In vivo expansion of HLA-B35 alloreactive T cells sharing homologous T cell receptors: Evidence for maintenance of an oligoclonally dominated allospecificity by persistent stimulation with an autologous MHC/peptide complex. J Exp Med 1995; 181:503-13.

65. Hand SL, Hall BL, and Finn OJ. T cell receptor Vβ gene usage in HLA-DR1-reactive human T cell populations: The predominance of Vβ8. Transplantation 1992; 54:357-67.

66. Geiger MJ, Gorski J, and Eckels DD. T cell receptor gene segment utilization by HLA-DR1-alloreactive T cell clones. J Immunol 1991; 147:2082-7.

67. Champagne E, Essaket S, Huchenq A, et al. Comparison of TCR-αβ sequences of cross-reactive anti-DR alloreactive T-cell clones: identification of possible contact residues based on charge complementarity between TCR chains and DR determinants. Eur J Immunogenetics 1992; 19:21-31.

68. Yamanaki K, Kwok WW, Mickelson EM, et al. T-cell receptor Vβ selectivity in T-cell clones alloreactive to HLA-Dw14. Human Immunol 1992; 33:57-64.

69. Goronzy J, Oppitz U, and Weyand CM. clonal heterogeneity of superantigen reactivity in human Vβ6+ T cell clones. Limited contributions of Vβ sequence polymorphisms. J Immunol 1992; 148:604-11.

70. Goronzy JJ, Xie C, Hu W, et al. Restrictions in the repertoire of allospecific T cells. J Immunol 1993; 151:825-36.

71. Wilson KE, Ball E, Stasny P, et al. Allorecognition of HLA DR2 and DR5 molecules by V-beta-8-positive T-cell clones. Scand J Immunol 1991; 33:131-9.

72. Beall SS, Lawrence JV, Bradley DA, et al. β chain rearrangements and Vβ gene usage in DPw2-specific T cells. J Immunol 1987; 139:1320-5.

73. Hansen T, Lundin KEA, Markussen G, et al. T cell receptor usage by HLA-DQw8-specific T cell clones. Int Immunol 1992; 4:931-4.

74. Liu Z, Sun YK, Xi YP, et al. Limited usage of T cell receptor Vβ genes by allopeptide-specific T cells. J Immunol 1993; 150:3180-6.

75. Liu Z, Sun YK, Xi YP, et al. T cell recognition of self-human histocompatibility leukocyte antigens (HLA)-DR peptides in context of syngeneic HLA-DR molecules. J Exp Med 1992; 175:1663-8.

76. Acha-Orbea H, Mitchell DJ, Timmerman L, et al. Limited heterogeneity of T cell receptors from lymphocytes mediating autoimmune encephalomyelitis allows specific immune intervention. Cell 1988; 54:263-73.

77. Urban JL, Kumar V, Kono DH, et al. Restricted use of T cell receptor V genes in murine autoimmune encephalomyelitis raises possibilities for antibody therapy. Cell 1988; 54:577-92.

78. Chluba J, Steeg C, Becker A, et al. T cell receptor β chain usage in myelin basic protein specific rat T lymphocytes. Eur J Immunol 1989; 19:279-84.

79. Waldmann TA. Immune receptors: targets for therapy of leukemia/lymphoma, autoimmune diseases and for the prevention of allograft rejection. Annu Rev Immunol 1992; 10:675-704.

80. Struyk L, Hawes GE, Chatilla M, et al. T cell receptors in rheumatoid arthritis. Arthritis Rheum 1995; In press.

81. Lehner PJ, Wang ECY, Moss PAH, et al. Human HLA-A0201-restricted cytotoxic T lymphocyte recognition of influenza A is dominated by T cell bearing the Vβ17 gene segment. J Exp Med 1995; 181:79-91.

82. Moss PA, Moots RJ, Rosenburg WM, et al. Extensive conservation of alpha and beta chains of the human T cell antigen receptor recognizing HLA-A2 and influenza A matrix peptide. Proc Natl Acad Sci USA 1991; 88:8987-90.

83. Bowness P, Moss PA, Rowland-Jones S, et al. Conservation of T cell receptor usage by HLA-B27-restricted influenza-specific cytotoxic T lymphocytes suggests a general pattern for antigen-specific major histocompatibility complex class I-restricted responses. Eur J Immunol 1993; 23:1417-21.

84. Hawes GE, Struyk L, Godthelp BC, et al. Limited restriction in the αβTCR V region usage of antigen specific clones: Recognition of myelin basic protein (a.a. 84-102) and Mycobacterium bovis 65kD heat shock protein (a.a. 3-13) by T cell clones established from PBMC of monozygotic twins and HLA identical individuals. J Immunol 1995; 154:555-66.

85. Wu CJ, Lovett M, Wong-Lee J, et al. Cytokine gene expression in rejecting cardiac allografts. Transplantation 1992; 54:326-32.

86. Stepkowski SM, Tu Y, Condon TP, et al. Blocking of heart allograft rejection by intercellular adhesion molecule-1 antisense oligonucleotides alone or in combination with other immunosuppressive modalities. J Immunol 1994; 153:5336-46.

T-CELL RECEPTOR USAGE AMONG GRAFT INFILTRATING T LYMPHOCYTES

James T. Kurnick, Makiko Kumagai-Braesch,
Carol P. Leary, Richard Waitkus, Lenora A. Boyle,
Peter J. van den Elsen and David M. Andrews

4. INTRODUCTION

Recognition of peptide-containing MHC molecules by the α/β T-cell receptor (TCR) has been shown to be the central controlling interaction which initiates specific cell-mediated immunity.[1,2] Although some stimuli, such as PHA and other polyclonal activators, can induce proliferation in virtually all T lymphocytes,[3] and "super antigens" can activate whole subsets of TCR-V region-selected T-cells[4], recognition of non-self MHC molecules (allo-antigens) remains the strongest truly antigen-specific stimulus yet described.[5-7] Thus, the rapid deployment of specifically-reactive T-cells to grafted allogeneic tissue and cells is a consistent feature of the immune response to allografts.

In vitro studies have indicated that up to several percent of circulating T-lymphocytes can recognize a given foreign MHC molecule. This cell-mediated response includes both CD4+CD8- MHC class II reactive T-cells, and CD4-CD8+ MHC class I reactive T-cells, which can recognize a myriad of peptides presented in the "groove" of these antigen-presenting molecules.[8] Not surprisingly, analysis of the T-cell receptor repertoire in response to these foreign MHC-peptide complexes shows extensive diversity both in TCRV gene segment usage and in the highly diverse CDR3 regions formed by the rearranged TCRV, D (β chain only) and J germ-line encoded and unique non-germline

The Human T-Cell Receptor Repertoire and Transplantation, edited by Peter J. van den Elsen. © 1995 R.G. Landes Company.

encoded N-nucleotides when the TCRAV-N-TCRAJ and TCRBV-N-TCRBD-N-TCRBJ segments rejoin to encode the "peptide" reactive elements of the αβ TCR.[9-11]

However, as attractive as it may be to purport that the in vitro Mixed Lymphocyte Reaction (MLR) is the true analog of in vivo alloantigen-recognition, there are several indications that the in vivo repertoire found within rejecting allografts represents only a fraction of the potential TCR repertoire. It is the finding of "preferred" T-cell receptor usage which will be the focus of this overview of our current understanding of the significance of TCR usage in allograft recognition.

4.1 Allograft-Infiltrating T Lymphocytes

It has been nearly 20 years since it was first demonstrated that rejecting allografts contain T lymphocytes capable of lysing donor target cells.[12,13] These cytotoxic allo-reactive T-cells were extracted directly from rejected kidney, and shown to be armed and ready to lyse cells bearing mismatched HLA antigens. In the intervening years, much has been learned about the true significance of the histocompatibility antigens, and the reason that these T-cell recognition structures are so strongly recognized as foreign, both in vivo and in vitro. The MLR proved extremely useful in demonstrating the ability of both the class II and class I MHC molecules to direct different components of cell-mediated immunity.[14] In addition to the now mature field of serotyping HLA antigens, using antibodies formed in response to paternal HLA antigens as a result of multiple pregnancies, the MLR and its cousin, the "Primed Lymphocyte Test" (PLT)[15,16] have helped to demonstrate both the diversity of the MHC antigens which can be found in a diverse ethnic population, but also the diversity of the T-cells able to respond to mismatched antigens.

More recently, the ability to investigate the role and spectrum of graft-infiltrating T lymphocytes (GITL) has been enhanced by methods which allow propagation of cells from even small tissue biopsies of still functioning grafts.[17-19] These in vitro culture methods have allowed a more comprehensive dissection of cell-mediated immunity in response to allogeneic tissues. As presaged by the studies of freshly isolated GITL, the IL-2 propagated cultures demonstrated both the intensity of MHC class I and II alloreactive T-cells, and the specificity towards donor antigens within the graft. Although it has long been recognized that circulating donor-specific cytotoxic T lymphocytes are rare, it has always been clear that strongly cytotoxic T-cells could be readily demonstrated within the graft. Furthermore, when multiple HLA antigen mismatches were known, it was usually easy to demonstrate reactivity to many, if not all mismatched class I and II HLA antigens. Not surprisingly, when cells were sorted or cloned, both proliferative and cytotoxic T-cells of both CD4+CD8- and CD4-CD8+ subsets could be demonstrated at strikingly high frequency.[20,21] Often more than half of the T-cell clones isolated from GITL showed donor-specific cytotoxicity or proliferation, or both, with CD4⁺CD8⁻ cells usually showing more intense proliferative activity and less cytotoxicity, and CD4⁻CD8⁺ cells showing generally more aggressive cytotoxicity and often less pronounced proliferation. However, T-cell clones of both phenotypes could be seen to show both activities simultaneously.[18,20,32]

All of these findings using GITL were consistent with what would be anticipated from the large number of in vitro studies using mixed lymphocyte reactions. However, a somewhat less expected finding emerged when studies began to focus on the TCR usage by various graft-infiltrating T lymphocytes.[17,22-27] As will be detailed in the following paragraphs, despite the finding that antigens recognized were often diverse, there began to mount increasing evidence for "favored" TCR usage in many GITL. Whether this selection at the site of alloantigenic stimulation represents the outgrowth of a few cells which have managed to "escape" the immunosuppression which allows graft survival, or a natural selection which can occur in many chronic inflammatory settings will be discussed in more detail below, as we attempt to summarize data from several settings, using differing technical approaches to determine if TCR selection is a feature of GITLs, and if so, how this selection arises and what it implies.

4.2 THE IN VITRO TCR RESPONSE

Before continuing the discussion of TCR use among GITL, we will briefly review TCR usage in mixed lymphocyte reactions. As noted, the MLR can be used to demonstrate both class II and I MHC mismatches,[28] and as this reaction proceeds in a matter of a few days (usually peaking at between 5 and 7 days), it would be anticipated that this assay would reveal much of the "potential" T-cell repertoire. Indeed, both the "precursor" frequency of proliferative and cytotoxic T-cells have been dissected extensively, with notable attempts to correlate these in vitro findings with behavior of host and graft in vivo; for example, in bone marrow transplantation, the CTLp has been discussed as one of the best predictors of graft acceptance and graft versus host disease (GvHD).[29,30]

As support for the notion of preferred TCR usage among allospecific T-cells, Suciu-Foca and colleagues demonstrated limited usage of T-cell receptor BV genes in the response of three individuals to a synthetic peptide corresponding to amino acid residues 21-42 of the DRB 1*0101 molecule.[31] In all three responders, reactivity to peptide 21-42 was restricted by the DR11 molecule, and all shared the expression of TCRBV13S2.

Among the first and most comprehensive studies of TCR usage among alloreactive T-cell T-cell clones was performed by Geiger, Gorski and Eckels[26] who studied the TCR usage among a group of HLA-

DR1-reactive T-cell clones. They noted diversity in TCRV gene usage among both TCR α and β chains and through analysis of amino acid sequences divulged some limitation in the CDR1 and 2 regions of different TCRV gene products. The CDR3 regions of the different T-cell clones were all very diverse, indicating heterogeneity among the "endogenous peptides" being recognized together with HLA-DR1 epitopes.

As will be discussed below for GITL, studies of TCR usage among allo-reactive clones serve to emphasize the enormity of the potential T-cell response. Not only is a major fraction of the T-cell said to be involved in recognition of even minor differences in MHC antigens, but when dissecting the TCR usage among clones reactive to a single class II MHC mismatch, HLA-DR, both diversity in TCRV gene segment usage, as well as diversity in the CDR3 region encoded by TCRAV-N-TCRAJ and TCRBV-N-TCRBD-N-TCRBJ, indicates that T-cells which recognize a given MHC alloantigen can be made up from widely divergent components of both α and β TCR chains, lending further credence to the polyclonal nature of the T-cell response to alloantigens. Thus, the findings to be discussed below that GITL are not as diverse as MLR-generated specific T-cells requires that mechanisms of in vivo selection be entertained to explain the appearance of favored clones and selected homologous CDR3 region structures.

4.3 ANALYSIS BY SOUTHERN BLOT

When the structure of the T-cell receptor genes and peptide chains began to be elucidated[32] after the cloning of the TCR β chain and then TCR α chain (as well as the TCR γ/δ chains[33]), a new means for evaluating T-cell repertoire was born. Although the TCRA gene structure does not make it amenable for analysis by Southern blotting, the TCRB gene structure[34] has proved to be quite fertile ground for determining if a T-cell "clone" is present within a population of T lymphocytes.[35-37] Based on the rearrangement of germline encoded TCRBV, TCRBD and TCRBJ genes to form a shortened TCRB gene configuration, it became apparent that certain restriction enzymes could be used to demonstrate T-cell receptor β gene rearrangement in distinction from the "germline" configuration of non-T lymphocytes. For example, the restriction endonuclease (EndoR) EcoR1 produces two germline products which hybridize with a TCRBC probe, indicative of the two germline TCRBC genes, either of which could be used in a productive rearrangement. An 11Kb fragment is formed in the germline as a result of cutting adjacent to the TCRBC1 gene, and a distinct 4Kb fragment formed to include the TCRBC2 gene. Virtually all T-cells would retain the 3' TCRBC2 gene, even if they rearranged to use TCRBC1, and all T-cells necessarily alter the germline configuration around the TCRBC1 fragment as it is either altered in rearrangement to TCRBC1, or lost if rearrangement occurs to TCRBC2. In similar fashion, rearrangements to TCRBC1 and TCRBC2 can be readily dissected using HindIII which proves particularly useful in exploring rearrangements to TCRBC2.

Used first to demonstrate T-cell malignancies,[35] it quickly became apparent that Southern blot analysis could also be used to demonstrate restricted T-cell receptor patterns among a variety of inflammatory conditions.[36] Initially applied in rheumatoid arthritis,[37] Southern blot analyses quickly found their way to the analysis of GITL.[17] Finn and colleagues demonstrated that GITL from kidney allografts were not as polyclonal as the in vitro MLR model might have predicted, and on repeat biopsies, the same "clonal" pattern of TCR usage could be demonstrated within the same patient.[17,23,24] In keeping with this finding, Frisman et al.[38] reported that serial cardiac allograft biopsies could be shown to demonstrate recurrent patterns of TCRβ chain gene rearrangements indicative of the persistence of a "favored" clone. An example of a recurrent rearrangement pattern as well as divergent rearrangements, are shown in Figure 4.1. Although these studies did not demonstrate the reactivity of the "dominant" T-cell clones, they did leave the distinct impression that GITL were not as diverse as one might have predicted.

Although Southern blotting of TCR genes has been purported to demonstrate T-cell clonal identity, the resolving power of such analyses does not always allow conclusive demonstration of true "clonality." Indeed, in a study of clones isolated from a kidney allograft, the "dominant" rearrangement which could be demonstrated among the "bulk" culture revealed clones of diverse origin, as each T-cell clone contained two rearranged TCRB genes, and the second rearrangement in each T-cell clone did not match the other.[38] As no DNA sequencing was performed in any of these early Southern blot analyses, the full implications of these data cannot be realized, but as will be discussed further below, the leads provided by these early studies remain valid, and several more recent studies confirm the strong possibility that GITL

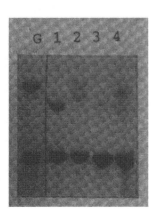

Fig. 4.1. Southern Blot analysis of GITL from serial myocardial biopsies from cardiac transplant. EcoR1 digest of DNA extracted from non T-cells (Germline = G) are shown in the first lane with the upper band of 11kb, and the lower band of 4kb. In lanes 1-4 are DNA digest from T-cells propagated from 4 different myocardial biopsies of a patient with several episodes of cellular rejection over a 2 year period. Each lane shows loss of the 11kb band and retention of the 4kb band. In lane 1 there is a non-germline band, and lane 4 a band which is different from the other biopsies. The GITL from biopsies 1 and 3 showed similar cytotoxic anti-graft HLA-specificity. GITL from biopsies 2 and 4 showed a different reactivity.

are not as diverse as the potential allo-repertoire, but do indeed represent a preferred T-cell infiltration.

4.4 ANALYSIS BY PCR

Study of TCR usage among-graft infiltrating T lymphocytes has also utilized PCR analyses using series of TCRAV and TCRBV specific oligonucleotide primer templates to detect possible skewed TCRV-gene usage. Among the several studies reported there are some common themes, and some disagreements, illustrated by the report of Hall and colleagues that the TCR repertoire among GITL became restricted over time in vitro, but the TCRBV repertoires of early GITL cultures were as heterogeneous as those of peripheral blood T lymphocytes (PBL).[24] They noted that both GITL and in vitro-derived MLR cultures became progressively more limited with respect to the TCRBV repertoire as they were expanded in vitro. They concluded that "functional subsets must be allowed to emerge from heterogeneous infiltrates before the TCR repertoire may be correlated with alloreactivity and/or graft rejection." These results put into perspective both the conclusions of the same group in a previous report using monoclonal antibodies and PCR which suggested a predominance of TCRBV8-bearing GITL among HLA-DR1-reactive T-cells.[23]

In other attempts to reveal TCR selection, the results were less conclusive. Krams et al.[39] suggested that TCRV gene usage among GITL was diverse, but that this might be a reflection of non-specific T lymphocytes which masked a possible selection among allo-specific GITL.[39] In a study from the Netherlands of GITL from serial myocardial biopsies, it was noted that individual biopsies contained GITL populations using different V region TCRs.[25] The T-cells analyzed from the serial biopsies indicated shifts in the TCRAV and TCRBV genes used from one biopsy to another, with some biopsies showing very limited TCRV gene usage. As myocardial biopsies often involve rather limited amounts of tissue with few infiltrating T lymphocytes, these results may reflect the small sample as well as a true shift in TCR repertoire. Of particular note, in one biopsy which showed strong allo-cytotoxic activity, multiple copies of a single graft-cytotoxic T-cell clone were sequenced and shown to use TCRBV20. A probe specific for the CDR3 region of this T-cell clone was used to determine if a previous biopsy, which also contained TCRBV20 transcripts that were indicative of the same clonotype, failed to detect this clone in the earlier specimen. These results suggested that the donor-specific cytotoxic T-cell clones had accumulated at the time of the rejection episode and were not present previously.[25]

Other studies have focused on bone marrow transplantation. In a study of graft versus host reactive T-cells which arose in the response of a Dw4 donor to a Dw14 host, a response which is due to a difference in only 2 amino acids, there was a suggestion that the specific T-cells show selective TCRV gene usage.[40] Although the T-cell cultures and T-cell clonings were done on in vitro primings from peripheral blood-derived T-cells, and consequently were not necessarily a reflection of the tissue-infiltrating T-cells, the TCR usage among these clones suggested recognition of highly conserved antigens by TCR with shared components. It must be noted that there is still considerable TCR heterogeneity among these clones, once again confirming the diversity of TCRs which can interact with a given MHC mismatch and the variety of peptides which can be presented by a given MHC molecule, but there is striking conservation of some CDR3 motifs in several of the clones indicating non-random patterns of TCR selection. For example, 20 of 42 clones used the TCRBJ2S7 gene segment, although N and TCRBD gene segment sequences were extremely heterogeneous. However, one feature in common to almost all of the observed TCRBJ gene segments was the presence of a negatively charged amino acid residue, either Glu or Asp in the CDR3, near the TCRVDJ junction in 93% of the sequences. However, when a second set of T-cell clones was prepared, the CDR3 sequences were not shared with those noted in the other T-cell cloning.[40]

Together these studies suggest that allografts can certainly contain a diverse array of specificities and diverse TCR, but that when one examines specific GITL which can be demonstrated in vitro, the repertoire does indeed indicate that preferred TCR structures do arise, indicating that these T-cell clones may have some selective in vivo advantage, related to their allo-antigenic specificity. Similar conclusions were drawn in an experimental rat allograft model.[27]

4.5 SPECTRATYPING AND SSCP

In addition to analyzing TCR usage by PCR, additional information may be acquired by studying the complexity of the CDR3 region diversity of a population of cells which share TCRAV or TCRBV gene expression. The enormous diversity of TCR usage is a product of the TCRV gene usage together with TCRBD (β chain only) and TCRJ region genes which recombine with the addition of random "N" nucleotides which gives the TCR repertoire its full diversity. In addition to sequencing an individual T-cell clone's α and β chains, or cloning the TCR genes into bacteria, it is possible to evaluate the extent of TCR-CDR3 diversity by two different methods: Spectratyping and Single Strand Conformational Polymorphism (SSCP).

Spectratyping, described by Gorski et al.,[22] allows one to determine if a population of T-cells with a given TCRAV or TCRBV have CDR3 regions of diverse, or restricted length. As productive recombinations must produce a CDR3 with multiples of three, allowing the rearranged genes to read in frame from TCRV through the TCRJ (and D for β) to TCRC regions, the distribution of PCR products provides a "ladder" of products, each differing by 3 nucleotides. Gorski et al.

used CDR3 spectratying to analyze the complexity and stability of circulating T-cell repertoires in normal adults, including bone marrow donors, and bone marrow transplant recipients. They demonstrated that normal spectratypes are both complex and stable. The TCR repertoire complexity of bone marrow recipients correlated with their state of immune function. Contractions and gaps in TCR repertoires were revealed in individuals suffering from recurrent infections associated with T-cell impairment. They noted that spectratype analysis is applicable to other studies of specific TCR repertoire skewing such as may be associated with immunodeficiency and that found at sites of immune activity.[22]

Another, somewhat more discriminating means of evaluating CDR3 heterogeneity involves the phenomenon of Single Strand Conformational Polymorphism (SSCP).[41] Unlike spectratyping which distinguishes only on the basis of CDR3 length, SSCP allows distinction of two different transcripts on the basis of nucleotide content and sequence, allowing detection of even a single nucleotide substitution in a product of several hundred bases. This technology is based on the differential electrophoretic migration of the individual complementary strands of a double-stranded PCR product, due to the difference in nucleotide composition of the two strands. After denaturation and electrophoresis on a non-denaturing gel system, the single stranded complementary strands of the PCR product adopt a unique folded conformation, based on nucleotide composition (sequence). This conformational polymorphism of the single strands of a PCR product leads to different migration rates through the non-denaturing gel. Under optimal conditions, SSCP technology can distinguish a single base pair difference in PCR products between 100 and 500 bases in length.[41] Therefore, this approach is well-suited for studying the diversity of the TCR structure, particularly for detecting differences in the CDR3 region at the TCRAV-TCRAJ and TCRBV-TCRBD-TCRBJ junctions. When a heterogeneous population of T-cells such as GITL is analyzed by SSCP, the electrophoretic banding pattern produced represents a "fingerprint" of the TCR usage for all T-cells in the population that transcribe that variable region.

Figure 4.2 shows an example of an SSCP analysis of T lymphocytes propagated from a patient whose longstanding myocarditis eventually led to a heart transplant. These heart-infiltrating T-lymphocyte populations were analyzed first by PCR with the whole spectrum of available TCRAV and TCRBV-family specific oligonucleotides, and a few TCRV region products which could be shown consistently among T lymphocytes isolated from serial biopsies (taken over a period of several years) were subjected to SSCP analysis. In this figure, the TCRBV2 products from several biopsy-derived T lymphocytes, and a peripheral blood sample, are shown. It can be seen that each specimen shows a distinctive banding pattern indicative of selection for individual T-cell clones in each specimen, but differences in the clonal pattern from one biopsy to the next. Although most of the specimens are from episodes of idiopathic myocarditis taken prior to transplantation, there are two specimens from the same patient taken after transplantation. Although the myocarditis specimens are quite distinctive, there is a faint doublet in the second transplant specimen which is similar to a doublet seen in the first transplant specimen. Sequence analysis will be necessary to determine if these specimens do indeed contain the same T-cell clone. However, in general, this analysis shows that the biopsies contain a few "clonal" T-cells, but are unique. No specificity for the cells corresponding to these TCR genes has been determined. However, there is evidence from SSCP analysis of T lymphocytes from arthritis patients[42] and T lymphocytes propagated from tumors (TIL) that, although each patient shows

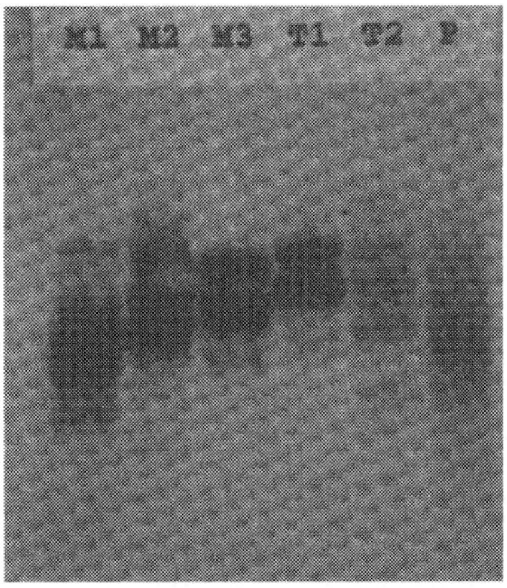

Fig. 4.2. PCR-SSCP analysis of T-cells propagated from myocardial biopsies. Infiltrating T lymphocytes from 3 serial biopsies from a patient with myocarditis were propagated in IL-2 and cDNA from these cultures were amplified in PCR using a $V\alpha2$-specific oligonucleotide primer. The $V\alpha2$ transcripts were then analyzed by SSCP. Lanes M1, M2 and M3 show different banding patterns from 3 different biopsies while the patient was suffering from myocarditis which eventually led to heart transplantation. Lanes T1 and T2 show a similar doublet banding among GITL propagated from two different post-transplant biopsies. Lane P shows the "smear" pattern seen in the polyclonal population of IL-2-responsive T-cells present in the peripheral blood of this patient post-transplant.

unique, selective TCR V region usage, there is extensive clonal dominance which can be appreciated even within T-cell populations.

For example, we analyzed a series of TCRAV2S1-expressing T-cell clones, and a bulk culture of TIL by SSCP. The SSCP "fingerprint" of these six T-lymphocyte clones showed three distinct patterns of migration, corresponding to three different N-TCRAJ sequences in these T-cell clones using the same TCRAV gene element. The bulk TIL propagated from this tumor biopsy showed a "dominant" doublet in the SSCP analysis corresponding to the position of bands from 3 of the T-cell clones which had identical TCRA sequences. One of these bands was cut, eluted, reamplified, and sequenced, and the sequence obtained matched perfectly with the TCRA of the three T-lymphocyte clones. The dominance of the SSCP TCR signal from these T-cell clones is consistent with these T-cells being present at high frequency in the bulk propagated TIL population (3 of 8 TCRAV2 clones obtained). Since the hybridization probe used in these analyses bound to the TCR constant region, the relative intensity of the electrophoretic bands is a reflection of their relative abundance in the T-cell culture from which the mRNA was extracted. Although SSCP is not suitable for analysis of individual TCR present in low frequency, the SSCP analysis for a given variable region family offers a fast, reproducible means for detecting clonal dominance in a population of T lymphocytes, and for comparing T-cell clones, as we have done for TIL.

4.6 ANALYSIS OF GRAFT-INFILTRATING T-CELL CLONES

While the majority of PCR and sequencing studies of GITL studies have focused on uncloned T-cell populations, we have evidence from analysis of several GITL clones that both selection for restricted HLA recognition, and shared TCR structures may play a role in response to allografts. In the study of 7 CD4+CD8- T-cell clones isolated from a brother-sister, single haplotype matched allograft, it was found that all of these CD4+CD8- T-cell clones reacted with the HLA-DR3 mismatch. The pattern of reactivity to the stimulator/targets from the 10th International Histocompatibility Workshop suggested that these T-cell clones were highly similar in their reactivity to HLA-DR3 epitopes in that all of them reacted with both the DR17 and DR18 splits of DR3, in distinction to most HLA-DR3 reactive clones from that workshop which recognized either DR17 or DR18, but not both.[43]

We chose to analyze these T-cell clones by PCR to determine the TCRV region gene usage for both the α and β chains, and to sequence the TCR transcripts from these T-cell clones to determine if there were shared motifs in their antigen-reactive moieties, particularly, the CDR3 region. Our results indicate that several different TCRAV and TCRBV gene segments are used among the different T-cell clones, but 2 of the T-cell clones that both kill and proliferate in response to HLA-DR3 share identical TCRAV27-TCRAJ-TCRAC and TCRBV13-TCRBD1-TCRBJ1S2-TCRBC1 transcripts as shown by sequencing. The additional 3 T-cell clones showed various TCRAV and TCRBV transcripts including one with TCRAV23, TCRAV16, TCRBV20; another with TCRAV4, TCRBV2 and TCRBV20; and the third with TCRAV7, TCRBV5A and TCRBV6. Although the TCRV regions usages were quite diverse, examination of the CDR3 regions of these T-cell clones indicated similarity in these antigen reactive sites of TCRB from 4 of the 5 T-cell clones. Analysis of the CDR3 regions of the TCRB reveals an intriguing sharing among these T-cell clones. As shown in Figure 4.3, the different TCRV regions use different TCRV gene products, but the CDR3 regions composed of the TCRBV-N-TCRBD-N-TCRBJ sequences resulted in amino acid sequences showing striking homology. For example, all 5 of the T-cell clones have aspartic acid (D) in the TCRBV-TCRBD-TCRBJ region, with some of the codons coming from germline TCRBD1, but others resulting from "N"

AMINO ACID SEQUENCES

antigen binding sites[1]

			----CDR3----			
			-V-	N-D-N	-J-	-C-
1A1	Db1.1	Jb 1.2	FCASS	**YDS**	HYGYTFGSGTRLTVV	EDLN
2D2	Db1.1	Jb 1.2	FCASS	**YDS**	HYGYTFGSGTRLTVV	EDLN
1c4	Db1.1	Jb1.5	LCAWS	**ERRDSG**	NQPQHFGDGTRLSIL	EDLN
2A9	Db2.1	Jb2.1	ICSA	**RDSGSS**	YNEQFFGPGTRLTVL	EDLK
2E10	Db1.1	Jb1.6	LCASS	**QDY**	NSPLHFGNGTRLTVT	EDLN

NUCLEOTIDE SEQUENCES

	N-BD-N	BJ
1A1 V13 (Db1.1 Jb1.2)	tac-gacag-c	cactatggctacacttcggttcggggaccaggttaaccgttgta
2D2 V13 (Db1.1 Jb1.2)	tac-gacag-c	cactatggctacacttcggttcggggaccaggttaaccgttgta
1C4 V20 (Db1.1 Jb1.5)	gaaagac-gggacag-cggc	aatcagcccagcatttggtgatgggactcgactctccatccta
2A9 V 2 (Db2.1 Jb2.1)	gctagagac-agcgggag-ttcc	tacaatgagcagttcttcgggccaggacacggctcacggtgcta
2E10V5a(Db1.1 Jb1.6)	-cagg-actat	aattcacccctccactttgggaatgggaccaggctcactgtgaca

1) Antigen binding sites are determined according to the reference of Chothia et al[44].
   Bold letters of amino acid sequence show the antigen binding sites.
2) Germ-line BD gene sequences are BD1.1 gggacaggggc, BD2.1 gggactagcgggaggg (Toyonaga et al.[45])

Fig. 4.3. Amino acid and nucleotide sequences of TCRBV D,J region.

region sequences entirely, or from a combination of germline TCRBD and "N" nucleotides, indicating the strong selective pressure for encoding of this amino acid. In four of the T-cell clones the amino acid adjacent to the aspartic acid is serine (S), which once again is encoded by a combination of TCRBD1 and "N" nucleotides in three T-cell clones, or by germline TCRBD2 in one instance. Additionally, 2 of the T-cell clones share an arginine-aspartic acid-serine amino acid sequence in this region, with "N" nucleotides contributing to RD sequences in both T-cell clones, and the S-residue being either germline or "N" encoded. Although both the CDR1 and CDR2 regions encoded by the TCRBV region genes are quite diverse among these T-cell clones, and there is additional N-TCRBD-N-TCRBJ diversity among the T-cell clones, it is clear that all 5 of the T-cell clones are reactive with the same HLA-DR3 molecule, and that there may also be shared epitopes on the "peptide" presented in the antigen groove, emphasizing selection for a limited antigen repertoire among T-cell clones of diverse origin.

These results suggest that although the repertoire for anti-HLA-DR3 reactive T-cell clones can include a diverse expression of TCRs, there may be a selective advantage for some T-cell clones (which appear in multiple copies), as well as conserved motifs in the CDR3 region of anti-DR3 specific T-cell clones, indicating immunodominant peptide epitopes in the antigen groove of this MHC molecule.

4.7 CONCLUSIONS

In this review we have attempted to summarize a variety of approaches to the evaluation of the T-cell repertoire in response to allografts. Although some conclusions remain undefined, there are several themes which can be summarized in the response to alloantigens in vitro and in vivo. First, it has long been apparent that the ability to respond to alloantigens includes a wide variety of T-cell subsets capable of responding to a multitude of mismatched alloantigens. Analysis of the TCR repertoire indicates no less diversity than was anticipated; there is diversity both in the usage of TCRAV and TCRBV genes, with extreme heterogeneity in the CDR3 regions, indicating that both the mismatched MHC antigens, and the processed peptides presented in the antigen "grooves" are heterogeneous, and the number of possible TCR combinations enormous.

With respect to allograft-infiltrating cells, the bottom line message which emerges is that the T-cell infiltrates are highly diverse if one evaluates all of the T-cells present within the graft. Although there are some reports which indicate some "selection" at the level of the TCR, this selection appears to reflect the antigen-specific component of the T-cell infiltrate, as non-specifically recruited cells almost certainly contribute to the total T-cell population present within rejecting allografts. However, one potentially important conclusion which is emerging from several studies is that the specific T-cell infiltrate may indeed show selection with respect to a few criteria.

There are several studies which indicate that multiple copies of the same T-cell clone may appear within inflamed tissues, including rejecting allografts, indicating that progeny of individual cells may have selective advantages in vivo. A more difficult to confirm conclusion suggests that there may also be preferred CDR3 configurations among the graft-specific T-cells, indicating that there may be some advantage to T-cells expressing some "preferred" antigen-recognition structures. Both the renal-allograft infiltrating T-cell clones we have described, and T-cell clones of graft-vs-host reactive T-cell clones isolated from the blood of a bone marrow transplant,[22] indicate preferred amino acids compose the peptide-recognizing structures in the CDR3 regions of many of the class II- MHC specific T-cell clones.

The results of the in vivo-activated alloreactive T-cell clones thus stands in contrast to the very diverse "potential" repertoire which can be readily demonstrated in vitro. The multiplicity of antigens which can be recognized remains diverse, and even in circumstances where selection can be demonstrated within an individual biopsy, subsequent biopsies appear to contain different T-cells with different TCR components, even when the mismatched antigens recognized are similar. These data demonstrate the resiliency of the immune response together with its enormous potential diversity. However, study of the T-cells infiltrating allograft tissues does reveal important selective pressures on the immune response to allo-antigens. The process of selection in the context of almost limitless potential diversity stresses the importance of studying how the immune repertoire is generated in vivo, not only in allografts, but in the myriad of inflammatory processes regulated by T lymphocytes.

ACKNOWLEDGEMENTS

This research was supported by grants NIH:HL-43793 and Nato (CRG 940029).

REFERENCES

1. Davis M and Bjorkman P. T-cell antigen receptor genes and T-cell recognition. Nature 1988; 334:395-402.
2. Marrack P and Kappler J. The antigen-specific, major histocompatibility complex-restricted receptor on T-cells. Adv Immunol 1986; 38:1-30.
3. Moretta A, Pantaleo G, Moretta L et al. Direct demonstration of the clongenic potential of every human peripheral blood T-cell-clonal analysis of HLA-DR expression and cytolytic activity. J Exp Med 1983; 157:743-54.
4. Kappler J, Kotzin B, Herron L et al. Vbeta-specific stimulation of human T-cells by staphylococcal toxins. Science 1989; 244:811-13.
5. Singal D. Quantitative studies of alloantigen-reactive human lymphocytes in primary and secondary MLC. Human Immunology 1980; 1:67-76.

6. Ryser J and MacDonald H. TI Limiting dilution analysis of alloantigen-reactive T lymphocytes. III. Effect of priming on precursor frequencies. Journal of Immunology 1979; 123:128-32.

7. Zhang L, Li S, Vandekerckhove B et al. Analysis of cytotoxic T-cell precursor frequencies directed against individual HLA-A and -B alloantigens. Journal of Immunological Methods 1989; 121:39-45.

8. Chien Y and Davis M. How alpha beta T-cell receptors 'see' peptide/MHC complexes. Immunology Today 1993; 14:597-602.

9. Danska J, Livingstone A, Paragas V et al. The presumptive CDR3 regions of both T-cell receptor α and β chains determine T-cell specificity for myoglobin peptides. Journal of Experimental Medicine 1990; 172:27-33.

10. Engel I and Hedrick S. Site-directed mutations in the VDJ junctional region of a T-cell receptor β chain cause changes in antigenic peptide recognition. Cell 1984; 54:473-84.

11. Patten P, Rock E, Sonoda T et al. Transfer of putative complementarity-determining region loops of T-cell receptor V domains confers toxin reactivity but not peptide/MHC specificity. Journal of Immunology 1993; 150:2281-94.

12. Tilney N, Garovoy M, Busch G et al. Rejected human renal allografts. Recovery and characteristics of infiltrating cells and antibody. Transplantation 1979; 28:421-26.

13. Von Willebrand E and Hayry P. Composition and in vitro cytotoxicity of cellular infiltrates in rejecting human kidney allografts. Cellular Immunology 1978; 41:358-72.

14. Meuer S, Schlossman S and Reinherz E. Clonal analysis of human cytotoxic T lymphcoytes: T4+ and T8+ effector T-cells recognize products of different major histocompatibility complex regions. Proc Natl Acad Sci USA 1982; 79:4395-99.

15. Zier K and Bach F. Secondary responses of human lymphocytes to alloantigens in vitro. Scandinavian Journal of Immunology 1975; 4:607-11.

16. Fradelizi D and Dausset J. Mixed lymphocyte reactivity of human lymphocytes primed in vitro. I. Secondary response to allogeneic lymphocytes. European Journal of Immunology 1975; 5:295-301.

17. Miceli MC and Finn OJ. T-cell receptor β-chain selection in human allograft rejection. J Immunol 1989; 142:81-86.

18. Mayer T, Fuller T, Lazarovits A et al. Characterization of in vivo activated allospecific T lymphocytes propagated from human renal allograft biopsies undergoing rejection. J Immunol 1985; 134:258-64.

19. Bonneville M, Moreau JF, Blokland E et al. T lymphocyte cloning from rejected human kidney allograft. Recognition repertoire of alloreactive T-cell clones. J Immunol 1988; 141:4187-95.

20. Preffer F, Colvin R, Leary C et al. Two color flow cytometry and functional analysis of lymphocytes cultured from human renal allografts: Identification of a Leu 2+3+ subpopulation. J Immunol 1986; 137:2823-30.

21. Stegagno M, Boyle L, Preffer F et al. Functional analysis of T-cell subsets and clones in human renal allograft rejection. Transplant Proc 1987; XIX:394-97.

22. Gorski J, Yassai M, Zhu X et al. Circulating T-cell repertoire complexity in normal individuals and bone marrow recipients analyzed by CDR3 size spectratyping. Correlation with immune status. J Immunol 1994; 152:5109-19.

23. Hand S, Hall B and Finn O. T-cell receptor V beta gene usage in HLA-DR1-reactive human T-cell populations. The predominance of V beta 8. Transplantation 1992; 54:357-67.

24. Hall B, Hand S, Alter M et al. Variables affecting the T-cell receptor V beta repertoire heterogeneity of T-cells infiltrating human renal allografts. Transpl Immunol 1993 1:217-27.

25. Datema G, Vaessen L, Daane R et al. Functional and molecular characterization of graft-infiltrating T lymphocytes propagated from different biopsies derived from one heart transplant patient. Transplantation 1994; 57:1119-23.

26. Geiger M, Gorski J and Eckels D. T-cell receptor gene segment utilization by HLA-DR1-alloreactive T-cell clones. J Immunol 1991; 147:2082-87.

27. Shirwan H, Chi D, Makowka L et al. Lymphocytes infiltrating rat cardiac allografts express a limited repertoire of T-cell receptor V beta genes. J Immunol 1993; 151:5228-38.

28. Dupont B, Hansen J and Yunis E. Human mixed lymphocyte culture reaction: Genetrics, specificity and biological implications. Adv Immunol 1976; 23:107-.

29. Batchelor J, Brookes P, Davey N et al. In vitro methods and selection of HLA-matched unrelated donors for bone marrow transplantation. Transpl Proc 1991; 23:1711-12.

30. Kaminski E, Hows J, Goldman J et al. Optimising a limiting dilution culture system for quantitating frequencies of alloreactive cytotoxic T lymphocyte precursors. Cellular Immunol 1991; 137:88-95.

31. Liu Z, Sun Y, Xi Y et al. Limited usage of T-cell receptor V beta genes by allopeptide-specific T-cells. J Immunol 1993; 150:3180-86.

32. Yanagi Y, Yoshikai Y, Leggett K et al. A human T-cell-specific cDNA clone encodes a protein having extensive hololology to immunoglobulin chains. Nature 1984; 308:145-49.

33. Haas W, Pereira P and Tonegawa S. Gamma/delta cells. Annual Reviews of Immunology 1993; 11:637-85.

34. Kronenberg M, Goverman J, Haars R et al. Rearrangement and transcription of the beta-chain genes of the T-cell antigen receptor in different types of murine lymphocytes. Nature 1985; 313:647-53.

35. Minden M, Toyonaga B, Ha K et al. Somatic rearrangement of T-cell antigen receptor gene in human T1 malignancies. Proc Nat Acad Sci USA 1985; 82:1224-27.

36. Weiss L, Wood G, Ellisen L et al. Clonal T-cell populations in pityriasis lichenoides et varioliformis acuta (Mucha-Habermann disease). Am J Pathol 1987; 126:417-21.

37. Stamenkovic I, Stegagno M, Wright K et al. Clonal dominance among T-lymphocyte infiltrates in arthritis. Proc Nat Acad Sci USA 1988; 85:1179-83.

38. Frisman DM, Hurwitz AA, Bennett WT et al. Clonal analysis of graft-infiltrating lymphocytes from renal and cardiac biopsies. Dominant rearrangements of TcR beta genes and persistence of dominant rearrangements in serial biopsies. Hum Immunol 1990; 28:208-15.

39. Krams S, Falco D, Villanueva J et al. Cytokine and T-cell receptor gene expression at the site of allograft rejection. Transplantation 1992; 53:151-56.

40. Yamanaka K, Kwok W, Mickelson E et al. Selective T-cell-receptor gene usage in allorecognition and graft-versus-host disease. Transplantation 1993; 55:1167-75.

41. Orita M, Suzuki Y, Sekiya T et al. Rapid and sensitive detection of point mutations and DNA polymorphisms using the polymerase chain reaction. Genomics 1989; 5:874-79.

42. Kitajima I, Yamamoto K, Sato K et al. Detection of human T-cell lymphotropic virus type I proviral DNA and its gene expression in synovial cells in chronic inflammatory arthropathy. Journal of Clinical Investigation 1991; 88:1315-22.

43. Kurnick J, Thomsen M, Irle C et al. T-Cell Recognition of HLA Class II Molecules. Chapter VII: DR3. Immunobiology of HLA, 1989.

44. Chothia C, Boswell DR, Lesk AM. The outline structure of the T-cell αβ receptor. EMBO J 1988; 7: 3745-55.

45. Toyanaga B, Yoshikai Y, Vadasz V et al. Organization and sequences of the diversity, joining and constant region genes of the human T-cell receptor β chain. Proc Natl Acad Sci USA 1985; 82:8624-28.

CHAPTER 5

T-Cell Receptor V-Gene Usage in T-Cell Lines Propogated from Graft-Infiltrating T Lymphocytes in Needle Biopsies of Rejecting Renal Allografts

Benito A. Yard, Thomas Reterink, Peter J. van den Elsen,
M.E. Paape, Jan Antony Bruijn, Leendert A. van Es,
Mohamed R. Daha and Fokko J. van der Woude

5. ABSTRACT

Needle biopsies taken from renal allografts of 42 renal transplant patients were tested for in vitro propagation of graft-infiltrating T-lymphocytes (GITL). From 30 out of 42 needle biopsies T-lymphocyte cell lines could be established. There was a significant correlation between in vitro outgrowth of T cells and histological signs of graft rejection. The majority of GITL cell lines displayed cytotoxicity both against donor proximal tubular epithelial cells (PTEC) and PHA stimulated donor splenocytes in an MHC class I restricted fashion. However, six cell lines were only cytotoxic against donor PTEC which is suggestive of recognition of tissue-specific antigens by these GITL derived T-cell lines. Analysis to the level of diversity of the T-cell receptor repertoire by PCR with TCRBV-family specific-oligonucleotides of a selection of these

The Human T-Cell Receptor Repertoire and Transplantation, edited by Peter J. van den Elsen. © 1995 R.G. Landes Company.

GITL derived cell lines revealed that the majority of the T-cell lines tested were polyclonal in nature on the basis of TCRBV gene family usage. A clear dominance of TCRBV genes was observed in only three GITL derived T-cell lines. There was no apparent correlation with the diversity of the TCRBV repertoire of GITL derived T-cell lines and the number of HLA-mismatches between the recipient and donor derived graft. Furthermore, the time interval between the transplantation and biopsy sampling did not contribute to the level of diversity of the TCRBV repertoire nor the tissue-specificity of these GITL derived T-cell lines.

5.1 INTRODUCTION

The hallmark of acute renal allograft rejection is generally accepted as injury to both endothelial and parenchymal cells, leading to impaired renal function. Although the exact mechanisms underlying renal allograft rejection are not fully understood yet, it is clear that alloreactive T cells play a key role in this process.[1,2] These alloreactive T cells may be involved in both initiation and maintenance of rejection.[3-5] This T cell allo-recognition might occur indirectly through presentation of donor derived peptides that are presented via recipient MHC class II molecules following capture by antigen presenting cells of the recipient or directly via recognition of donor derived MHC/peptide complexes.[6,7] These various recognition events result in the activation and proliferation of alloreactive T cells that may mediate graft destruction directly.[8] Mononuclear cells of recipient origin usually infiltrate the renal allografts. These graft-infiltrating T lymphocytes (GITL) often show donor specific cytotoxicity in vitro. The presence of these allograft-infiltrating T cells does not necessary result in acute allograft rejection.[9,10] T-cell lines from percutaneous needle biopsies performed on renal transplant patients during rejection episodes can be established in vitro in the presence of IL-2.[11-13] Outgrowth of these graft-infiltrating T lymphocytes is correlated to histological signs of graft-rejection.[13-15] In most cases these allograft-derived T-cell lines exhibit cytolytic activity against various types of donor derived target cells.

The immunological rejection process in renal allo-transplantation is primarily the consequence of differences between the donor and the recipient in the expressed components of the major histocompatibility complex (MHC) which includes the pool of "self"-peptides presented by the MHC. In acute rejection periods mono-nuclear infiltrates can easily be detected after cadaveric renal transplantation in humans even under adequate immunosuppression.[16] As a result of damage to both endothelial and parenchymal cells the allografted kidney becomes functionally impaired.

During the process of renal allograft rejection expression of intercellular adhesion molecule 1 (ICAM-1) is induced de novo on renal tubular cells.[17,18] Expression of MHC class II antigens may also be induced by cytokines produced by inflammatory cells.[19,20] Proximal tubular epithelial cells (PTEC) may possibly present antigen and thus function as accessory cells, as suggested by the capacity to express ICAM-1, MHC class II molecules and the production of costimulatory factors such as tumor necrosis factor α (TNFα) and IL-6.[21] Histological signs of tubular damage by graft-infiltrating T-lymphocytes correlates with significant clinical rejection, as has been shown previously.[18] Moreover in vitro studies suggested that PTEC may function as a target during renal allograft rejection.[22]

There are several lines of evidence which suggest that in the process of antigen recognition by T cells the complexes formed by MHC and peptide are capable of selecting T-cell receptor α and β chains which optimally fit their target structure.[23-26] Both in the MHC class I and II system restrictions in the responding T-cell receptor repertoire have been reported.[27-32] Therefore, studies in renal transplantation were initiated on the premise that clonal expansion of T cells in the allograft could serve as a target for specific immune interventions on the basis of inactivation or elimination of the presumed pathogenic T cells.

We have studied the nature of graft-infiltrating T-lymphocyte cell lines propagated from kidney needle biopsies during rejection episodes with respect to T-cell receptor V-gene family usage. This was done to determine whether these in vitro established T-cell lines exhibited a restricted character of TCRBV gene family diversity which would be indicative of an alloresponse directed against a dominant alloantigen.

5.2 MATERIALS AND METHODS

PATIENTS

We have included in this study 14 patients selected from a group of 42 patients who had received a renal allograft. The HLA types of the selected patients and donors are depicted in Table 5.1. The majority of these patients received a kidney obtained from a postmortal donor. The group of patients was treated with prednisone in an initial dose of 20 mg/day tapered in steps of 2.5 mg/2 weeks to 10 mg/day, and cyclosporine A 10 mg/kg/day tapered to 5 mg/kg/day in three months. Dosage adjustments were made according to serum levels. Patients who received a haplo-identical kidney from a living related donor, had received a donor specific transfusion and were treated with the same immunosuppressive therapy as the recipients of cadaveric kidneys.

CELL CULTURE

For the isolation of graft infiltrating T lymphocytes (GITL) small tissue fragments were put in a 24 well plate containing "Iscove's" Modified Dulbecco's Medium (IMDM) in the presence of 5% T-cell growth factor (TCGF) and 10% fetal calf serum (FCS). After a period of 2 weeks, during which the medium was refreshed 3 times, outgrowing T cells were pooled, seeded in a concentration of $0.2.10^6$ cells/ml in a 24 well plate and polyclonally restimulated with irradiated (300 rad), peripheral

Table 5.1. Cultured GITL from renal allografts: HLA-typing of donor and recipient, sex, age, histology, time interval between biopsy and transplantation and cell surface phenotype of cells by FACS

Patient	Sex/age	Type of the HLA donor	Type of the HLA recipient	Time interval [a]	TBM [b]	Graft loss	Histological evaluation	CD3	CD4	CD8	WT31
1	F/33	A1 B8 CW7 DR3	A1 A29 B8 B14 DR2 DR3	72	+	+	Severe int.[c] rej. severe vasc.[d] rej.	98	52	38	100
3[E]	M/54	A26 A29 B5 BW22 DR4 DR5	A2 A29 B5 B12 DR4 DR5	24	±	+	Severe int. rej. severe vasc. rej.	99	78	25	90
4	F/52	A2 B27 DR4	A2 A24 B7 B27 DR4 DRW53	7	+	·	Severe int. rej.	97	43	62	93
5	M/50	A2 A3 B7 B18 CW7 DR2 DR3	A2 A3 B7 B18 CW7 DR2 DR3	74	+	-	Moderate int. rej.	100	25	70	96
6[E]	F/52	A1 A2 B7 B8 CW7 DR2 DR3	A2 B7 B44 CW5 CW7 DR2 DR5	52	+	+	Severe vasc. rej.	98	18	80	89
8	F/42	A1 A3 B14 B37 CW6 DR3 DR4	A3 B7 B27 CW2 CW7 DR3 DR4	8	-	+	Diffuse clotting, no rejection	100	64	42	95
9	M/42	A2 A31 B51 B44 CW4 CW5 DR5 DRW8	A2 A3 B16 B35 CW4 DR5 DRW8	7	±	·	Slight int. rej.	97	40	53	96
12	M/64	A1 A29 B8 B12 DR3 DR5	A1 B8 B17 DR3	6	+	+	Moderate int. rej.	98	87	13	93
15	M/45	A2 B5 B60 CW4 CW6 DRW6 DRW13	A2 B5 B60 CW4 CW6 DRW6 DRW13	9	+	+	Severe int. rej.	99	14	82	88
17[E]	F/23	A1 B5 B17 DRW6 DR7	A2 AW19 B12 B15 DR4 DRW8	75	+	+	Severe int. rej. severe vasc. rej.	97	27	76	96
18[E]	M/37	A1 A2 B7 B8 DR3 DR4	A1 A2 B7 B8 DR3 DR4	67	+	+	Severe int. rej. severe vasc. rej.	96	47	61	92
19	M/26	A2 A3 B5 DR1 DR2	A11 A29 B5 BW53 DR1 DR2	7	-	·	Slight int. rej.	99	92	10	97
21	M/65	A3 A31 B44 B27 CW2 CW5 DR4	A2 A29 B45 B27 CW2 CW6 DR4	164	±	+	Moderate int. rej. severe vasc. rej.	99	54	49	92
22	M/53	A2 A3 B18 B35 CW4 DR1 DR5	A2 A28 B44 B14 CW5 DR4	8	-	·	Slight int. rej.	98	50	45	99

a Interval between biopsy and transplantation in days
b Tubular basement membrane damage
c Interstitial rejection
d Vascular rejection
E Material obtained by transplantectomy

blood mononuclear cells (PBMC) (10^6 cells/ml) and OKT3 ($1:10^5$ from ascites). T cells were restimulated once a week. Every 3 or 4 days the medium (IMDM with 10% FCS and 5% TCGF) was refreshed.

GITL were in eight cases isolated from kidneys obtained by transplantectomy. In all other cases GITL were isolated from biopsies. PTEC were isolated according to the protocol of Detrisac et al.[33] Briefly, small tissue fragments were put on a matrix of collagen (Vitrogen Sigma, St. Louis, MO, U.S.A.) and FCS, in culture flasks. After 30 minutes at room temperature, the culture medium was gently put into the flasks. The medium used was serum free DMEM/HAM F12 in a ratio of 1:1 supplemented with insulin (5 µ/ml), transferrin (5 µg/ml), selenium (5 ng/ml), hydrocortisone (36 ng/ml), triiodothyronine (4 pg/ml) and epidermal growth factor (EGF, all from Sigma). Usually after 3 weeks of primary culture, monolayers of PTEC were tryprisized passaged into other flasks and cultured in the above mentioned medium.

Biopsies were only done on clinical grounds. For this investigation one extra puncture (18 gauge Biopty®-system, Sweden) was performed during the biopsy procedure under echographic guidance. The exact time intervals between transplantation and biopsy are given in Table 5.1. This study was approved by the Medical Ethics Committee of the University Hospital Leiden, and informed consent was obtained from all patients. Donor lymphocytes were isolated from the spleen and stimulated with PHA 0.1 µg/ml (Sigma, St. Louis, MO, U.S.A.) in IMDM supplemented with 10% FCS and 5% TCGF.

CHARACTERIZATION OF PTEC
AND PHENOTYPING OF GITL LINES

PTEC were characterized by binding of a monoclonal antibody (MoAb) directed against the epithelial membrane antigen (EMA, Dakes, Glostrup, Denmark) and two other MoAbs (1071 and 1072) directed against adenosine deaminase binding protein (kindly provided by Dr. Dinjens, University Hospital, Maastricht, The Netherlands). Phenotyping of GITL T-cell lines was performed by FACS analysis. Staining was done by a two step immunofluorescence technique using MoAbs directed against CD3 (OKT3), CD4 (OKT4), CD8 (OKT8) and TCR α/β (WT31), (all from ATCC, Rockville, MD, U.S.A.) as first antibody followed by a goat anti-mouse FITC conjugated IgG (Becton and Dickinson).

CYTOTOXICITY ASSAY

Cytotoxicity was measured using a standard ^{51}Cr release assay. Briefly, target cells were labeled with 100 µCi of ^{51}Cr for 1 hour at 37°C in humidified air with 5% CO_2. After washing twice 5.10^3 labeled cells were put in each well of a 96 well plate (U bottom Costar, Cambridge, MA, U.S.A.) containing 4 different concentrations of effector cells (total volume 200 µl). The plate was centrifuged (1200 rpm, 5 min) and incubated further for 4 hours at 37°C in humidified air with 5% CO_2. Thereafter the plate was centrifuged again and 100 μl of each well was harvested and counted in a gamma counter. In each experiment, for each target a medium control and a Triton X-100 control was included.

Specific ^{51}Cr release was calculated by the formula:

$$\% \text{ specific release} = \frac{\text{CPM sample - CPM medium x 100\%}}{\text{CPM Triton X-100 - CPM medium}}$$

Blocking experiments were performed with anti-HLA class II (B8.11,2 a gift from Dr. M. Giphart, Department of Immunohematology and Blood Bank, University Hospital Leiden, The Netherlands), anti-HLA class I (W6/32), anti-CD3 (OKT3), anti-CD4 (OKT4), anti-CD8 (OKT8) and anti-CD18 (IB4) (all from ATCC, Rockville, MD, U.S.A.) in an ascites dilution of 1:100. Antibodies were present during the assay.

RNA ISOLATION, PCR AMPLIFICATION
AND CHARACTERIZATION OF THE PCR-AMPLIFIED PRODUCT

Total RNA was isolated from approximately 10^7 T cells by extraction with RNAzol (Cinna/Biotecx-Laboratories, Houston, TX, U.S.A.). Five μg of total RNA was converted into first strand cDNA using oligo dT primers according to the manufacturer's instructions (Promega Corporation, Madison, WI, U.S.A.). PCR amplification and Southern blot analysis were essentially the same as described by Lambert et al.[34] or by Struyk et al.[35]

STATISTICAL ANALYSIS:
Statistical analysis of 2 x 2 contingency tables was done using a chi-square test.

5.3 RESULTS

FUNCTIONAL CHARACTERIZATION
OF ALLOGRAFT DERIVED T-CELL LINES

From 30 out of 42 biopsies done on clinical grounds, we were able to generate T-cell lines as described in the materials and methods section. There was a highly significant correlation between the outgrowth of T cells and the histological finding of rejection (p = 0.0014, Table 5.2).

There were 5 patients who suffered from rejection, but no in vitro outgrowth of T cells from the biopsy was achieved. Only in 1 patient who did not suffer from rejection, outgrowth of T cells could be observed (Table 5.2). In biopsies from patients suffering from moderate to severe interstitial rejection, damage of the tubular basement membrane (TBM) could be detected.

Table 5.2. In vitro outgrowth of T cells from biopsies of renal transplant patients with and without interstitial rejection

n = 42	Rejection	No rejection
Outgrowth	29	1
No outgrowth	5	7

TBM damage in the biopsy was not correlated to the outgrowth of T cells cytotoxic to proximal tubular epithelial cells.

T-cell lines from 25 different donor recipient combinations were subsequently studied for cytotoxicity against donor target cells. Four T-cell lines could not be studied. The outgrowth of cytotoxic T cells from biopsies could thus be tested in 38 patients and was significantly correlated (p < 0.001) to the presence of interstitial rejection (Table 5.3).

Of these 25 different GITL derived T-cell lines, 14 donor recipient combinations were selected for further studies. All of these GITL-derived T-cell lines expressed the αβTCR and in the majority of cases were of a mixed CD4⁺CD8⁻/CD4⁻CD8⁺ phenotype (Table 5.1). These T-cell lines displayed various levels of cytotoxicity against donor target cells. T-cell lines from patients 1 and 12 did not manifest cytotoxicity against donor derived PTEC nor PHA-blasts, whereas for instance T-cell lines from patients 6 and 9 displayed cytotoxicity both against PTEC and PHA-blasts. The GITL-derived cell lines from patients 3, 4 and 5 only lysed donor derived PTEC since no lysis was observed with donor derived PHA-blasts. Treatment of PTEC with IFN gamma for 72 hours to upregulate adhesion molecules and MHC class I and induction of MHC class II, did not necessarily result in an increased susceptibility to lysis (e.g. patients 1, 3, 4, 6, 9, Table 5.4). However, there were two GITL derived T-cell lines (from patients 19 and 21, Table 5.4) that showed a clear increase in cytotoxicity against IFN gamma treated PTEC.

Table 5.3. Cytotoxicity against IFN gamma treated PTEC by cultured GITL cell lines from biopsies of renal transplant patients with and without interstitial rejection

n = 38	Rejection	No rejection
Cytotoxicity	20	0
No cytotoxicity	10	8

Table 5.4. Cytotoxicity of patient GITL cell lines against: a; donor PTEC cultured in plain medium, b; donor PTEC cultured in medium supplemented with 200 U/ml of IFN gamma for 72 hours

Patient	PTEC Medium[a]	IFN gamma[b]	PHA blasts
1	9	3	5
3	44	35	0
4	27	28	0
5	13	25	0
6	74	68	60
8	41	68	ND
9	33	36	12
12	0	0	ND
15	6	15	ND
17	11	24	100
18	10	23	ND
19	9	73	42
21	7	26	ND
22	43	64	ND

In addition cytotoxicity was tested against PHA blasts. Cytotoxicity is expressed as mean % specific ^{51}Cr release.

Table 5.5

Patient no.	Medium	Anti-CD3	Anti-CD4	Anti-class II	Anti-CD8	Anti-class I	Anti-CD18
3	37	5	28	31	21	15	2
4	38	1	41	38	18	8	6
5	23	9	·ND	27	16	18	14
6	35	7	38	35	23	17	ND
8	57	6	55	59	14	12	5
9	32	5	29	27	15	13	11
17	24	3	27	25	8	7	4
19	73	12	42	37	65	67	12

Results are expressed as mean % of specific ^{51}Cr release. All MoAb were used in ascites dilution of 1:100 and were present during the assay

The nature of the lysis against IFN-gamma treated PTEC lines was investigated further (Table 5.5). In all cases the cytolytic activity of the GITL-derived cell lines could be inhibited with antibodies against CD3 and CD18. The blocking activity of the monoclonal antibodies shows that both the TCR/CD3 mediated signaling pathway and the LFA-1/ICAM-1 adhesion pathway are crucial factors in the cytolytic activity of the GITL. In GITL derived from patient 19, the inhibition of cytolytic activity with antibodies against CD4 and MHC class II suggest that the cytolytic activity is carried by the CD4+CD8- T cells which predominate in this cell line (Table 5.1). In most other GITL the cytolytic activity is MHC class I restricted.

TCRBV GENE REPERTOIRE
OF RENAL ALLOGRAFT-INFILTRATING T-LYMPHOCYTE DERIVED CELL LINES

A number of T lymphocyte cultures established from graft-infiltrating T-lymphocytes of renal allografts were subjected to analysis of TCRBV gene usage. These GITL derived T-cell lines were chosen on the basis of HLA (haplo)-identity and disparity between the donor and the recipient and the level of cytotoxicity of these T-cell lines. The results of these analyses were compared to paired samples of peripheral blood mononuclear cells (PBMC) taken at the same time of the biopsy and cultured in a similar fashion as the T-cell lines from the biopsy (only 1 PBMC derived T-cell line is shown). The TCRBV repertoire of peripheral blood lymphocytes in these renal allograft patients shows an extensive usage pattern of TCRBV gene families. This suggests that the combinatorial diversity in these transplant patients is similar to normal controls (see chapter 2). Consequently the immunosuppressive drugs these patients were taking at the time of sampling had no major influence on the overall composition of the peripheral TCRBV repertoire on the basis of TCRBV gene family usage. In most of the T-cell lines analyzed, multiple TCRBV families could be detected (Figs. 5.1 and 5.2). Only in the cell lines propagated from the needle biopsies of patients 12, 15 and 19 a restricted pattern of TCRBV family usage was noted. There was no apparent correlation to the number of HLA mismatches between the donor and recipient, since in three HLA matched (haplo)-identical cadaveric donor recipient combinations a broad TCR repertoire was also found (patients 1, 3, 4, 5 and 6, Figs. 5.1 and 5.2) whereas in the three cell lines with a TCRBV dominance only in one case the T-cell line was generated from a patient who received an HLA matched identical cadaveric graft (patient 15, Fig. 5.1).

TCRBV dominance also did not correlate with the time interval between biopsy and transplantation since polyclonality was seen in GITL derived T-cell lines generated from biopsies taken already 7 days after transplantation (T-cell lines from patients 4 and 9, Figs. 5.1 and 5.2). Severity of rejection was not associated with a polyclonal character of the T-cell line generated from the biopsy. For example, the T-cell line from patient 9 with slight interstitial rejection was polyclonal, whereas the T-cell line from patient 15 with severe interstitial rejection was oligoclonal (Table 5.1, Figs. 5.1 and 5.2).

5.4 DISCUSSION

There is evidence derived from several studies which suggests that there is a significant correlation between the in vitro outgrowth of T cells from renal biopsies and the occurrence of rejection.[13] Furthermore, there is an apparent correlation between rejection and outgrowth of T cells in conjunction with cytotoxicity of the graft-infiltrating T cells.[13-15] In most cases this cytotoxicity was MHC class I restricted.

Analysis of the nature of the renal allograft infiltrating T-lymphocyte repertoire has revealed that αβ T cells predominate. Depending on the culture conditions for the propagation of graft-infiltrating T-lymphocytes, T-cells carrying the αβ T-cell receptor could also be found among such cultures.[36] In our study, all the in vitro established T-cell lines from renal allograft infiltrating T lymphocytes expressed the αβ T-cell receptor. Analysis to the level of combinatorial diversity of the αβ T-cell receptor revealed that in general, multiple TCRBV families could be detected among the graft-infiltrating T lymphocytes, with the exception of 2 T-cell lines. Whether this apparent restricted character indeed represents a clonal expansion of T lymphocytes in the renal allograft biopsies, needs further investigation.

The outcome of the character of the T lymphocyte repertoire of tissue-infiltrating T lymphocytes also depends on the initial cell number in the biopsy. Since these transplant patients were selected for kidney needle biopsies because of renal malfunction, which is the direct consequence of severe tissue-damage related to mononuclear cell infiltration into the allograft, it seems feasible to assume that the cell numbers were abundant. As shown in the cardiac transplant model[37] there seems to be an apparent correlation between the severity of the rejection and the cell numbers of graft-infiltrating T lymphocytes. In several biopsies there was no apparent correlation between the number of TCRBV families detected in T lymphocyte cell lines propagated from kidney needle biopsies and the severity of the rejection. However, taking into consideration that the graft-infiltrating T lymphocytes are unevenly distributed in the allograft during rejection, the sampling might have influenced the outcome of these analyses.

Although the cell lines propagated from the needle biopsies exhibited cytotoxic activity in vitro, the diversity of the T lymphocyte repertoire at the clonal level has not been determined. Hall and Finn[38] have shown that allo-reactive cytotoxic T-cell lines with known speci-

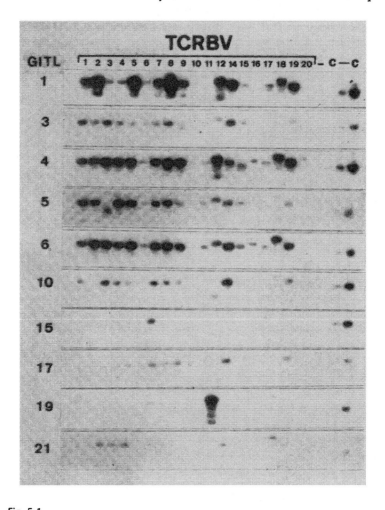

Fig. 5.1

ficity propagated from kidney needle biopsies exhibited a paucity in the number of gene elements used in the makeup of the TCRBV-regions. Furthermore, their observation that the initial immune response in the graft is oligoclonal and later becomes polyclonal suggest that non-specific T lymphocytes are attracted to the allograft as a result of the inflammatory process which results in tissue damage and eventually failure in graft-function and rejection.[39] This non-specific invasion might obscure the initial restriction in the effector immune repertoire. Bonneville et al.[36] have shown the polyclonal nature of the graft-infiltrating T lymphocytes from a rejection kidney obtained by transplantectomy from a patient who had been without immunosuppression for 14 days. Similarly, the level of diversity of the T lymphocyte repertoire of transplantectomised kidneys in our studies was always extensive suggesting that in these rejected organs multiple T cells have been attracted to the site of rejection.

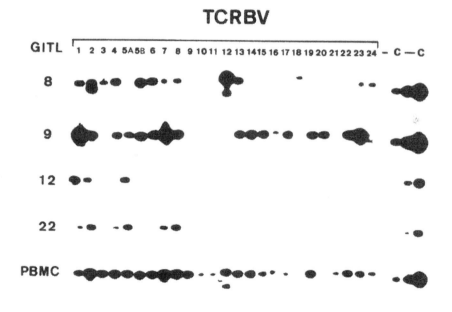

Fig. 5.2

Figs 5.1 and 5.2. Southern blot analysis of the PCR products of TCRBV-gene family specific amplification by PCR of GITL derived T cell lines propagated from kidney needle biopsies. The PCR products were electrophoresed and transferred to the nylon membranes as described (Lambert et al.[34]; Struyk et al.[35]). TCR β chain specific nucleotide sequences were detected by hybridization with a TCRBC-specific probe. Lanes 1-20 (or 1-24) represent the individual TCRBV-gene family specific oligonucleotides used in the PCR amplification, (-) represents the water control and C-C represents 1:5, 1:25 and 125 serial dilutions of the TCRBC internal control amplification.

Taking into consideration the number of HLA mismatches, there was no apparent correlation between the diversity of the unselected T lymphocyte repertoire and the number of HLA mismatches of the donor and recipient. A similar observation was also made by Krams et al.[40] who studied T-cell receptor α and β chain expression in nephrectomies and kidney needle biopsies. In freshly isolated tissue-samples they observed general usage of multiple TCRAV and TCRBV gene families and no apparent correlation between the number of TCR families represented and the number of HLA mismatches.

As shown in Figures 5.1 and 5.2, T-cell lines generated from HLA-matched identical cadaveric donor recipient combinations exhibited a polyclonal character (see also Table 5.1). As discussed above this is most likely the direct consequence of the ongoing rejection process which attracts non-specific T lymphocytes to the site of inflammation.

The results of the T-cell receptor V gene usage of unselected renal allograft infiltrating T lymphocytes have shown extensive usage of both TCRAV and TCRBV gene families.[40-42] Hall and Finn, however, have provided evidence that among established allospecific T-cell lines, the T-cell receptors expressed by these allospecific T-cell lines exhibited a more restricted nature of T-cell receptor V gene usage.[38] Following in vitro establishment of T-cell lines from renal allograft infiltrating T lymphocytes, the initial cultures were usually polyclonal. In T-cell lines which exhibited either anti-MHC class II (anti-DR) or anti-MHC class I (anti HLA-A,B) reactivity, the T-cell receptor repertoire became more restricted upon prolonged in vitro culture and stimulation with donor Epstein Barr virus (EBV) transformed B-lymphocytes.

Taken together, the results of these various studies suggest that an analysis of the allo-specific T-cell receptor repertoire of graft-infiltrating T lymphocytes might reveal T-cell receptor specificities which exhibit a more restricted character of combinatorial diversity of T-cell receptor α and β chains. Given the fact that the number of T-cell receptor V gene family specific monoclonal antibodies is increasing, the restricted nature of the T-cell receptor allo-specific repertoire might allow for a more specific immune intervention during allograft rejection.

ACKNOWLEDGEMENTS:
    This study was supported by the Dutch Kidney Foundation (Grant no. C88812).

REFERENCES
    1. Hall BL and Dorsch SE. Cells mediating allograft rejection. Immunol Rev 1984; 77:31-60.
    2. Mason DW. Effector mechanisms in allograft rejection. Ann Rev Immunol 1986; 4:119-45.
    3. Rosenthal AS and Shevach EM. Function of macrophages in antigen recognition by guinea-pig T lymphocytes: II. Role of macrophages in the

regulation of genetic control of the immune response. J Exp Med 1973; 138:1213-17.

4. Ziegler K and Unanue ER. Identification of a macrophage antigen processing event required for l-region-restricted antigen presentation to T lymphocytes. J Immunol 1981; 127:1869-75.

5. Wood PJ and Streilein JW. Immunogenetic basis of required transplantation tolerance. Transpl 1984; 37:223-26.

6. Matzing P, Bevan MJ. Hypothesis: Why do so many lymphocytes respond to major histocompatibility antigens? Cell 1977; 29:1-5.

7. Bevan MJ. High determinant density may explain the phenomenon of alloreactivity. Immunol Today 1984; 5:128-30.

8. Hall BL. Cells mediating allograft rejection. Transpl 1991; 51:1141-51.

9. Versluis DJ, Ten Kate FJW, Wenting GJ et al. Mononuclear cells infiltrating kidney allograft in the absence of rejection: effect of conversion from cyclosporine to azathioprine therapy. Transpl Int 1988; 1:205-08.

10. Ouwehand AJ, Vaessen LMB, Baan CC et al. Alloreative lymphoid infiltrates in human heart transplants: loss of class II directed cytotoxicity more than 3 month after transplantation. Hum Immunol 1991; 30:50-59.

11. Mayer TG, Fuller AA, Fuller TC et al. Characterization of in vivo-activated allospecific T lymphocytes propagated from human renal allograft biopsies undergoing rejection. J Immunol 1985; 134:258-64.

12. Miceli MC, Metzgar RS, Chedid M. Long-term culture and characterization of alloreactive T-cell infiltrates from renal needle biopsies. Hum Immunol 1985; 14:295-304.

13. Kirk AD, Ibrahim MA, Bollinger RR et al. Renal allograft-infiltrating lymphocytes. A prospective analysis of *in vitro* growth characteristics and clinical relevance. Transpl 1992; 53:329-38.

14. Bollinger RR, Miceli C, Finn OJ, et al. Monitoring the donor-specific response of renal transplant patients by needle biopsy and long term culture of alloreactive T-cell clones. Transpl Proc 1986; 18:748-49.

15. Miceli MC, Barry TS, Finn OJ. Human allograft-derived T-cell lines: Donor class I- and class II-directed cytotoxicity and repertoire stability in sequential biopsies. Hum Immunol 1988; 22:185-98.

16. Mac-Whinnie DC, Thompson JF and Taylor HM. Morphometric analysis of cellular infiltration assessed by monoclonal antibody labeling in sequential human renal allografts. Transpl 1986; 42:352-58.

17. Bishop GA, Hall BL. Expression of leukocyte and lymphocyte adhesion molecules in the human kidney. Kidney Int 1989; 36:1078-85.

18. Moolenaar W, Bruijn JA, Schrama E et al. T-cell receptors and ICAM-1 expression in renal allografts during rejection. Transpl Int 1991; 4:140-45.

19. Pastelnak MS. Cytotoxic T lymphocytes. Adv Intern Med 1988; 33:17-44.

20. Bishop GA, Hall BL, Suranyi MG et al. Expression of HLA antigens on renal tubular cells in culture. I. Evidence that mixed lymphocyte culture supernatants and gamma interferon increase both class I and class II HLA antigens. Transpl. 1986; 42:671-79.

21. Yard BA, Daha MR, Kooymans-Couthino M et al. Il-1α stimulated TNFα production by cultured human proximal tubular epithelial cells (PTEC). Kidney Int 1992; 42:383-84.

22. Van der Woude FJ, Daha MR, Miltenburg AMM et al. Renal allograft-infiltrated lymphocytes and proximal tubular cells: Further analysis of donor-specific lysis. Human Immunol 1990; 28:186-92.

23. Engel I, Hedrick SM. Site-directed mutations in the VDJ junctional region of a T-cell·receptor β chain cause changes in antigenic peptide recognition. Cell 1988; 54:473-84.

24. Sorger SB, Paterson Y, Fink PJ et al. T-cell receptor junctional regions and the MHC molecule affect recognition of antigenic peptides by T-cell clones. J Immunol 1990; 144:1127-35.

25. Danska JS, Livingstone AM, Paragas V et al. The presumptive CDR3 regions of both T-cell receptor α and β chains determine T cell specificity for myoglobin peptides. J Exp Med 1990; 172:27-33.

26. Jorgensen JL, Esser U, Fazekas de St.Groth B et al. Mapping T-cell receptor-peptide contacts by variant peptide immunization of single-chain transgenics. Nature 1992; 355:224-30.

27. Acheo-Orbea H, Mitchell DJ, Timmermann L et al. Limited heterogeneity of T-cell receptors from T lymphocytes mediating autoimmune encephalomyelitis allows specific immune intervention. Cell 1988; 54:263-73.

28. Hedrick SM, Engel I, McElligott DL et al. Selection of amino acid sequences in the beta chain of T-cell antigen receptor. Science 1988; 239:1541-44.

29. Gold DP, Offner H, Sun D et al. Analysis of T-cell receptor β chains in Lewis rats with experimental allergic encephalomyelitis: conserved complementarity determining region 3. J Exp Med 1991; 174:1467-76.

30. Moss PA, Moots RJ, Rosenberg WM et al. Extensive conservation of α and β chains of the human T-cell antigen receptor recognizing HLA-A2 and influenza A matrix peptide. Proc Natl Acad Sci 1991; 88:8987-90.

31. Van Schooten WCA, Long Ko J, Van der Stoep N et al. T-cell receptor β-chain gene usage in the T-cell recognition of Mycobacterium leprae antigens in one tuberculoid leprosy patient. Proc Natl Acad Sci 1992; 89:11244-48.

32. Bowness P, Moss PA, Rowland-Jones S et al. Conservation of T-cell receptor usage by HLA B27-restricted influenza-specific cytotoxic T lymphocytes suggests a general pattern for antigen-specific major histocompatibility complex I-restricted responses. J Immunol 1993; 23:1417-21.

33. Detrisac JC, Sens MA, Garvin AM et al. Tissue culture of human kidney epithelial cells of proximal origin. Kidney Int 1984; 25:383-90.

34. Lambert M, Van Eggermond M, Mascart F et al. TCRVα and β gene segment usage in T-cell subsets derived from a tye III bare lymphocyte patient deficient in MHC class II expression. Dev Immunol 1992; 2:227-36.

35. Struyk L, Kurnick JT, Hawes GE et al. T-cell receptor V-gene usage insynovial fluid lymphocytes of patients with chronic arthritis. Human Immunol 1993; 37:237-51.

36. Bonneville M, Moisan JP, Moreau JF et al. TCR alpha, beta and gamma gene rearrangements in human alloreactive T-cell clones extracted from a rejected kidney. Transpl Proc 1988; 20:196-98.

37. Datema G, Vaessen LMB, Daane RC et al. Functional and molecular characterization of graft-infiltrating T lymphocytes propagated from different biopsies derived from are heart transplant patient. Transpl 1994; 57:1119-26.

38. Hall BL and Finn OJ. T-cell receptor Vβ gene usage in allograft-derived cell lines analyzed by a polymerase chain reaction technique. Transpl 1992; 53:1088-99.

39. Micelli MC, Barry TS and Finn OJ. T-cell receptor β-chain selection in human allograft rejection. J Immunol 1989; 142:81-86.

40. Krams SM, Falco DA, Villanueva JC et al. Cytokine and T-cell receptor gene expression at the site of allograft rejection. Transpl 1992; 53:151-56.

41. Yard BA, Kooymans-Couthino M, Reterink T et al. Analysis of T-cell lines from rejecting renal allografts. Kidney Int 1993; 43, suppl. 39:133-38.

42. Hall BL, Hand SL, Alter MD, Kirk AD and Finn OJ. Variables affecting the T-cell receptor Vβ repertoire: Heterogeneity of T-cell infiltrating human renal allografts. Transpl Immunol 1993; 1:217-27.

======= CHAPTER 6 =======

STRUCTURE OF T CELL RECEPTOR Vα AND Vβ CHAINS EXPRESSED BY T-LYMPHOCYTES IN CARDIAC ALLOGRAFT DERIVED CELL LINES

Gert Datema, Len Vaessen, Rene Daane, Carla Baan,
Willem Weimar, Frans Claas and Peter van den Elsen

6. SUMMARY

Cellular rejection of a cardiac allograft is mediated by T-lymphocytes. To study the function of these T cells, graft infiltrating T-lymphocytes propagated from endomyocardial biopsies were analyzed for their capacity to lyse donor derived target cells. Subsequently, the structure of T cell receptor V-regions was analyzed to determine the nature of the cardiac alloresponses. Our studies have revealed that donor-specific cytotoxic T cell lines can be established from endomyocard-infiltrating T-lymphocytes. T cell clones established from these donor-specific T cell lines displayed multiple specificities against donor encoded cell surface antigens. Some of these allo specific T cell clones expressed identical T cell receptors, revealing that they were derived from the same progenitor. T cell clones specific for different donor allo-antigens expressed multiple TCRAV and TCRBV regions. Also, T cell clones, reactive against the same donor allo-antigens, but established from sequentially taken biopsies from the same patient displayed a different TCRAV and TCRBV repertoire. Taken together,

The Human T-Cell Receptor Repertoire and Transplantation, edited by Peter J. van den Elsen. © 1995 R.G. Landes Company.

our studies suggest that within a given patient the allo-specific T cell repertoire of T cells which have accumulated into the cardiac allograft is compressed.

6.1 INTRODUCTION

Heart transplantation is now a common surgical procedure for the treatment of several end-stage cardiac diseases. However due to the nature of these transplants, which include in almost all cases HLA mismatched donor-recipient combinations, the major complication in cardiac transplantation is acute rejection. The diagnosis of rejection after clinical heart transplantation is based on histologic criteria. Therefore endomyocardiac biopsies (EMB) are taken at regular intervals after transplantation. The histological rejection grade in heart transplantation is assessed according to the Billingham criteria[1]: Grade 0, no evidence of rejection, no visible mononuclear cell infiltrate; Grade 1, mild rejection, diffuse perivascular and endocardial infiltration with pyroninophilic lymphocytes, endocardial and interstitial edema; Grade 2, moderate rejection, more dense perivascular, endocardial and interstitial infiltration with pyrorinophylic lymphocytes, and focal myocytolysis (necrosis); grade 3, severe rejection, vessel wall and myocyte necrosis with interstitial bleeding, interstitial infiltrates with polymorphonuclear cells and pyroninophilic lymphocytes; grade 4, resolving rejection, active fibrosis, some small nonpyroninophilic lymphocytes, some plasma cells and hemosiderin.

The immunological mechanisms that mediate allograft rejection are not yet fully understood, but it is well established from both experimental and clinical transplantation that T-lymphocytes play an important role in the initiation and mediation of allograft rejection.[2,3] Graft-infiltrating T-lymphocytes can easily be detected via morphometric techniques[4] and it is possible to propagate graft-infiltrating T-lymphocytes from allograft tissue by in vitro cell culture.[5,6] The specific function of these graft-infiltrating T-lymphocytes (GITL) in the complex network of allorecognition and rejection is not clear. It is assumed however that these graft-infiltrating T-lymphocytes participate in the regulatory and effector stage of the immune response since activated T cells have been identified and expanded from rejecting human allografts.[7] The majority of T cells that infiltrate the allografted heart express the αβ T cell receptor and is composed of both CD4+CD8- and CD4-CD8+ T cells. Among these CD4+CD8- and CD4-CD8+ graft-infiltrating αβ T-lymphocytes T-cells can be found that are capable of recognizing specific MHC class I and class II mismatches on donor-derived Epstein-Barr Virus transformed B cell lines (B-LCL).[7-11]

T cell activation is initiated following specific recognition by the T cell receptor (TCR) of MHC molecules and/or complexes formed by MHC and antigenic peptides on the antigen presenting cell (APC). Within the TCR α and β chains the so called complementarity determining regions (CDR) are directly involved in contacting the MHC/peptide complex.[2,12-15] The CDR 1 and 2 are comprised within the TCR V genes whereas the CDR3 region is the direct product of the TCRV, (TCRD), TCRJ joinings. There are several lines of evidence which suggest that the CDR3 region interacts with the peptide presented by the MHC. In this regard it was shown in various studies that modifications in the CDR3 region of the TCR affects the recognition of the MHC/peptide complex.[15,16] Moreover the amino acid composition of the presented peptide seems to direct the composition of amino acids in the CDR3 loops of TCRs.[17,18] In a number of studies involving specific antigenic peptides both in the MHC class I as well as MHC class II system it was found that in humans the MHC/peptide complex mediated selection of TCR V regions. These studies showed restricted TCR V gene usage and shared amino acid motifs in the CDR3 regions by TCRs of T cells specific for the given MHC/peptide complexes.[19-25] These observations suggest that MHC/peptide complexes are able to select for TCR V regions that optimally fit their counterstructures. In this light, selective accumulation and expansion of T-lymphocytes can be determined through analysis of TCR V regions of graft-infiltrating T-lymphocytes in comparison to similar analysis of paired samples of peripheral blood derived T-lymphocytes.

To determine the nature of the alloresponse in heart-transplant patients with respect to the level of clonality of the responding T-lymphocytes and whether in the alloresponse T cell receptors use specific TCR V genes and CDR3 regions, we have performed a number of studies both at the functional and molecular level. For these studies T-lymphocytes were propagated from endomyocard biopsies and were analyzed for T cell receptor V-gene usage and structure of the TCRV α and Vβ chains. Where possible the studies were performed in relation to function.

6.2 MATERIALS AND METHODS

6.2.1 PATIENTS AND BIOPSIES
HLA-class I and -class II typing of the patients (PATA, PATB and PATC) and their donors used in this study are tabulated in Table 6.1. In all cases, patients received a preoperative blood transfusion and were transplanted with HLA-mismatched donor hearts. All patients received immunosuppressive drugs (Cyclosporin A and a low dose of prednisone). Endomyocardial biopsies (EMB) were taken according to protocol. In the first 6 weeks posttransplant at weekly intervals, the next 4 weeks every 2 weeks, once every 4 weeks up to 18 weeks, from 18 to 30 weeks once in 6 weeks and between 30. and 52 weeks posttransplant an EMB was taken once in 2 months, declining to once every four months more than one year after heart transplantation. After an acute rejection episode the next biopsy was taken

Table 6.1 HLA-class I and -class II typing of the three donor/recipient combinations used in this study

	HLA-A	HLA-B	HLA-C	HLA-DR
PATA	2,11	35,62(15)	3,4	4,-
donor	1,29(19)	8,44(12)	7,-	3,15(2)
PATB	1,3	7,8	7,-	3,-
donor	2,11	60(40),62(15)	1,3	1,4
PATC	2,3	7,57(17)	3,4	1,7
donor	1,2	8,62(15)	3,7	1,13(6)

one week following rejection therapy. During right ventricular catheterization four or five biopsy samples were obtained. Of these EMB samples, three to four were used for histological evaluation and one was used for the propagation of the T cell infiltrate. Administration of rabbit antithymocyte globulin (RATG) or corticosteroids was given as rejection therapy when rejection grade 2 was observed.

6.2.2 GENERATION OF T CELL LINES FROM EMB

Each biopsy of PATA and PATB was divided into 2 fragments and each placed in two wells of a 96 well U-bottom tissue culture plate (Costar 3799, Cambridge, MA, U.S.A.) with 200 µl culture medium in the presence of 10^5 irradiated (30 Gy) autologous PBMC as feeder cells. Culture medium (CM) consisted of RPMI-1640-Dutch modification (Gibco, Paisley, Scotland) supplemented with 10% v/v lectin-free Lymphocult-T-LF (Biotest GmbH, Dreieich, FRG) as exogenous source of IL-2, 10% pooled human serum, 4mM L-glutamine, 100 IU/ml penicillin and 100 µg/ml streptomycin. The CM for the biopsy fragments of PATA and PATC was supplemented with 0.1 µg/ml PHA (Wellcome).

PBMC were isolated by Ficoll-Isopaque (δ = 1.077) density gradient centrifugation. Biopsy cultures were grown at 37°C in a humidified atmosphere with 5% CO_2.

For PATA propagated T-lymphocytes from one of the biopsy fragments were, after 8 days of culture, further expanded by restimulation with random PBMC and third party B-LCL until sufficient cells were obtained for analysis (32 - 70 days). The graft-infiltrating T lymphocyte (GITL) cultures obtained in this way were considered as bulk cultures.

For PATB every 2-3 days half of the medium was replaced by fresh CM. When cell growth was observed the wells were pooled and further expanded when sufficient cell density was reached (10^5 – 10^6 cells/ml).

After three weeks of culture, when growth was slowing down or cell death was observed the cultures of PATB were restimulated by adding 5.10^3/well irradiated (30 Gy) EBV transformed third party B cells (B-LCL) until enough cells were obtained for analysis.

For PATC and the other half of the biopsy fragment, the second well, of PATA the biopsy fragment was removed after two days of incubation. The GITL were seeded over 96 wells of a microtitre plate (Costar) with CM, and 10^5 (irradiated) random PBMC and 5.10^3 (irradiated) third party B-LCL as feeders, this culture was called GITL day 2 culture (GCD2). The biopsy fragment was washed to remove adhering cells and cultured for another two days in the presence of irradiated autologous PBMC and third party B-LCL in CM with 0.1µg/ml PHA. After two days the biopsy fragment was removed again and the propagated GITL day 4 (GCD4) were seeded over 96 wells, similar as described for day two. This procedure was repeated two times more (GCD6 and GCD8). After ten days of culture no more T cells could be propagated from the biopsy fragment. Two weeks after restimulation of the mini bulk cultures GCD2, GCD4, GCD6 and GCD8, the number of growing wells was determined. Growing wells were split in two, and restimulated with random PBMC and third party B-LCL in CM. This procedure was repeated every 2 weeks untill 8 daughter, mini-bulk cultures, were obtained from every original well. Those mini-bulk cultures were phenotyped and assayed for cytotoxicity against donor B-LCL, third party B-LCL and K562.

6.2.3 GENERATION OF T CELL CLONES

Randomly stimulated GITL cultures of PATA and PATB were washed and cloned by limiting dilution at 0.3 cells per well in a 96 well U-shaped tissue culture plate in 200 µl culture medium containing 0.1 µg PHA and 20 U/ml rIL-2 in the presence of 10^5 irradiated (30 Gy) random feeder cells and 10^4 irradiated (50 Gy) B-LCL. After 10-14 days the growing cultures were transferred to a 24 well plate (Costar) and restimulated with PHA and rIL-2 in the presence of third party B-LCL and random PBMC.

6.2.4 MONOCLONAL ANTIBODIES

Cultured cells were phenotyped by flow cytometry using 1.10^5 cells for each labeling. The following purified, PE or FITC labeled monoclonal antibodies (mAb) were used: anti-Leu-2 (anti-CD8), anti-Leu-3 (anti-CD4), anti-Leu-4 (anti-CD3) and WT31 (anti-αβTCR) (Becton Dickinson, Mountain View, CA, U.S.A.). βV5a (anti-TCRBV5S2/3), βV5b (anti-TCRBV5S3), βV6 (anti-TCRBV6S7), βV8 (anti-TCRBV8), βV12 (anti-TCRBV12), αV2 (anti-TCRAV2S3), αV12 (anti-TCRAV12) (T Cell Sciences, Inc. Cambridge, MA, U.S.A.) and TCRBV2S1, TCRBV3S1, TCRBV5S1, TCRBV8S1, TCRBV13S6, TCRBV17S1, TCRBV18S1 (Immunotech, Marseilles, France). Inhibition studies were performed using the following mAb: W6/32 and B1.23.2 (both directed against monomorphic HLA class I structures),[26] B1.1G6 (anti-β_2-microglobulin),[27] PdV5.2 (directed against a monomorphic epitope shared by DR, DP and most of the DQ alleles),[28] WT32 (anti-CD3),[29] FK18 (anti-CD8)[30] and RIV6 (anti-CD4, RIVM, Bilthoven, The Netherlands).

6.2.5 CYTOTOXICITY ASSAY

Four daughter plates of the four seeding points (GCD2, GCD4, GCD6, GCD8) from each growing biopsy of patients PATA and PATC were used.

To two plates 3.10^3 ^{51}Cr-labeled donor B-LCL were added. The 2 other plates were used to determine the specificity of the cytotoxicity, therefore one plate was incubated with 3.10^3 ^{51}Cr-labelled third party B-LCL (different from the one used for restimulation) and one with 3.10^3 ^{51}Cr-labelled K562 as a control on lymphikine activated killer cells (LAK) and natural killer (NK) activity of the cultures.

The plates were centrifuged (600 g, 1 min) and incubated for 4 hours at 37°C in a humidified atmosphere with 5% CO2.

Supernatants were collected with a Skatron harvesting system (Skatron-AS, Lierse, Norway) and counted in a gamma counter for 3 minutes. From each well the % lysis was calculated according to the formula:

$$\% \text{ lysis} = \frac{\text{experimental release - spontaneous release}}{\text{maximal release - spontaneous release}} \times 100$$

Maximal release was determined in six-fold from a Triton X100 (5% v/v solution in 0.01 M TRIS-buffer) lysate of the target cells. Spontaneous release was determined in six-fold, by incubation of target cells in medium (RPMI-1640-Dutch modification, supplemented with 1% heat inactivated human serum) only.

The mean lysis % was then determined for the two corresponding wells. Mini-bulk-cultures that lysed donor target for more than 10% and did not show activity against third party and K562 were considered positive.

The bulk cultures from all three patients were assayed for cytotoxicity as follows:

A total of 2.10^4 effector cells (T cell lines or T cell clones) were mixed with 2.10^3 ^{51}Cr-labeled target cells (B-LCL) in 200 µl medium (RPMI-1640-Dutch modification, supplemented with 1% heat inactivated human serum) in U-shaped microtiter wells. The plates were centrifuged (600 g, 1 min) and incubated for 4 hours at 37°C in a humidified atmosphere of 5% CO$_2$. The supernatants were harvested using a Skatron harvesting system and counted in a gamma counter. Percentage of lysis was calculated as described previously.[31] Inhibition of cytotoxic activity with mAb was carried out as follows: an appropriate dilution of the mAb containing ascites was preincubated with 2.10^3 target cells or 2.10^4 effector cells in 0.1 ml medium at 37°C. After 30 minutes 2.10^4 effector or 2.10^3 target cells were added without prior washing of the preincubated cells.

6.2.6 RNA EXTRACTION AND TRANSCRIPTION

Cultured T-lymphocytes (5 to 10.10^6) were purified by centrifugation through a Ficoll Isopaque gradient. Following washing with HBSS (Gibco, Paisley, Scotland) the cells were pelleted by centrifugation and stored at -70°C for the molecular analyses. Total RNA was extracted using the RNAzol method (Cinna/Biotecx, Laboratories Inc, Houston, TX, U.S.A.). 5µg of total RNA was transcribed into first strand cDNA in 25 µl reaction mixture by reverse transcriptase using oligo dT as a primer (Promega Corporation, Madison, WI, U.S.A.).

6.2.7 PCR AMPLIFICATION

TCR α and β chain encoding cDNAs were amplified by using 22 or 28 different TCRAV and 19 or 25 different TCRBV family specific oligonucleotides using the methodology as described by Hawes et al.[32] For these polymerase chain reactions 0.5-1.0 µl of cDNA was added to a PCR mixture containing 10 mM Tris-HCl pH 8.4, 50 mM KCl, 4 mM $MgCl_2$, 0.06 mg/ml BSA, 0.5 mM of each dATP, dCTP, dGTP and dTTP, 2.5 units of Taq DNA polymerase (Boehringer, Mannheim, FRG), 20 pmol of a TCR 3' C-region primer and 20 pmol of a TCR V-family specific 5' primer in a final volume of 100 µl. As an internal control for total amplification, a reaction tube containing a 3' and 5' C-region primer was included. The sequences of these primers were derived from Lambert et al.,[33] Wucherpfennig et al.,[19] Oksenberg et al.[34] and Hawes et al.[32] Each reaction mixture was overlaid with 50 µl of mineral oil (Sigma, St. Louis, MO, U.S.A.) prior to PCR reaction in a thermal cycler (Biomed, Thermocycler 60). TCRAV and TCRBV specific sequences were amplified for respectively 30 and 25 cycles. Each cycle consisted of 1 min denaturation at 95°C, 1 min annealing at 55°C and 1 min extension at 72°C.

6.2.8 DETECTION AND QUANTIFICATION

PCR products were size fractionated by electrophoresis on 1% agarose gels in Tris-acetate/EDTA buffer, visualized by staining with ethidium-bromide and in case of PATA subsequently transferred to nylon membranes (Biotrace, Gelman Sciences, Ann Arbor, MI, U.S.A.). TCRAV and TCRBV specific sequences were detected by hybridization with ^{32}P-labeled TCRAC or TCRBC probes respectively according to the Biotrace protocol. Autoradiograms were analyzed by densitometry (LKB 2220-020, Ultrascan XL, Laser Densitometer, Pharmacia LKB Biotechnology, Uppsala, Sweden) to measure the intensity of the bands. To achieve a relative value for the amount of amplification the densitometry values were normalized with respect to the C-region internal controls of the GITL and PBMC as follows:

$$\text{measured V gene family intensity} \quad X \quad \frac{\text{measured C gene intensity of PBMCPATA.0}}{\text{measured C gene intensity}}$$

6.2.9 DNA CLONING AND SEQUENCING

5' TCRAV or TCRBV and 3' TCRAC or TCRBC sequence specific primers were used to generate PCR products from the T cell clones and the EMB derived T cell lines PATA.4 and PATA.5. PCR products of PATA were purified through Qiagen columns (Diagen GmbH, Düsseldorf, FRG). The purified PCR products and Sma I digested pUC 19 plasmids were tailed with dATP and dTTP respectively (Boehringer, Mannheim, FRG). dA-tailed PCR products were ligated into the dT-tailed pUC 19 plasmids overnight at 16°C and subsequently transfected into E.coli JM101. Positive colonies were expanded, purified through Qiagen columns, and the DNA sequence was determined by using the T7 DNA Polymerase Sequencing System (Promega Corporation, Madison, WI, U.S.A.). PCR products of patient PATB were size fractionated by low melting agar and subsequently purified using PCR 'Wizard' columns (Promega, Madison, WI, U.S.A.). The DNA sequence of the purified PCR products was determined by using the Circumvent Thermal Cycle Dideoxy DNA Sequencing Kit (New England Biolabs, Beverly, MA, U.S.A.). The sequencing products were resolved on polyacrylamide gels and detected by autoradiography.

6.2.10 CDR3 DETECTION

To detect the presence of allo-specific TCR β-chain sequences an oligonucleotide was synthesized on the basis of the CDR3 sequence as detected in the HLA-A29 specific T cell clones of PATA. This TCR β chain CDR3 oligo (5'-CATAAGCAGGCCCTACACTC-3') was labeled with [32]P γATP and used for detection of homologous sequences by hybridization of TCRBV20 family specific PCR products in the PATA.4, PATA.5 and PBMC derived PATA T cell lines.[35]

6.3 RESULTS

To elucidate the T cell-mediated mechanisms involved in allograft rejection, we have performed functional and molecular studies on T lymphocytes infiltrating the endomyocardium after cardiac transplantation from three different individuals. For these studies endomyocardial biopsies, sequentially taken before, during and after a histologically determined rejection episode, were used. T lymphocyte cell lines, both bulk cultures and mini-bulk-cultures were established (see Materials and Methods), phenotyped, and assessed for their cytolytic capacity against donor B-LCL and/or B-LCL sharing 1 or more HLA antigens with the donor B-LCL.

6.3.1 PROPAGATION CHARACTERISTICS OF THE GITL CULTURES

From the EMB of PATA and PATC mini-bulk cultures were established every two days, to obtain information about the time necessary to propagate donor specific T cells from the biopsy. From Table 6.2 it is evident that despite the presence of a polyclonal T cell mitogen very few GITL cultures could be established from the first three EMB of PATA. Although most of the mini-bulk cultures contained predominantly CD8 positive TCR-αβ T cells, non of them showed cytotoxic activity against donor antigens. Although, for PATC (Table 6.3) 59 of the 96 day 2 subcultures of the first EMB (PATC-1GCD2) contained αβ T cells, only 2 of them displayed donor directed cytotoxicity.

For the EMB with myocytolysis (grade 2), EMB5 for PATA, and EMB3 for PATC, essentially the same pattern of outgrowth was observed. From the mini-bulk cultures initiated 6 and 8 days after culture onset of the EMB, all 96 wells contained T cells and most of them were cytotoxic against donor derived B-LCL (Table 6.2 and 6.3). The mini-bulk cultures established from these rejection biopsies on day 2, from PATA (5GCD2) 45% of the wells contained T cells and from PATC (3GCD2) 76% of the wells. However only 1 resp 3 minicultures were cytotoxic for donor cells. From the on day four established cultures of those rejection biopsies (5GCD4 and 3GCD4), a smaller number of wells (± 30%) had T cells when compared to the previous point. However, 30% of the wells contained donor directed cytotoxic T cells. Unfortunately, due to infection in the mini cultures, PATC-3GCD4 cultures could not be assessed for cytotoxicity. This relation between increase in the number of wells with T cells cytotoxic for donor antigens and later propagation time was for PATA also observed for the biopsy preceding the rejection biopsy (EMB4, Table 6.3).

Although both patients, after successful rejection treatment with RATG, did not encounter a second acute rejection period, growth and cytotoxicity patterns were remarkably different.

From the biopsies 7 and 8 of PATA growing cultures could not be established and none of the mini-bulk cultures derived from the biopsies 6 and 9 showed donor directed cytotoxicity (Table 6.2).

For PATC (Table 6.4) the situation was completely different: from all biopsies up to 232 days post transplantation (EMB12) T cell cultures could be established, mostly at high frequency. The majority (93%) of the cultures (4GCD2-8) obtained from the biopsy directly preceding RATG treatment, were not cytotoxic for donor antigens. This was also the case for the EMB9 and EMB11 (Table 6.3). EMB5 showed another pattern than the other biopsies in that most cultures with cytotoxic T cells were now found in the first mini-bulk (5GCD2, Table 6.3) instead of cultures which were started later as seen for the EMB 6,7,8,10 and 12 (Table 6.3).

Table 6.2. PATA

HIST[1]	EMB minibulk	Growth #[2]	Phenotype WT31CD4[+] #[3]	Phenotype WT31CD8[+] #[3]	Phenotype WT31CD4[+] WT31CD8[+4]	Donor specific CML #[5]
1	1GCD2	1		1		0
	1GCD4	2		1		0
	1GCD6	0				
	1GCD8	0				
1	2GCD2	2	1	1		0
	2GCD4	0				
	2GCD6	3		3		0
	2GCD8	0				
1	3GCD2	1		1		0
	3GCD4	1		1		0
	3GCD6	3	2	1		0
	3GCD8	0				
1	4GCD2	27	10	15*		1
	4GCD4	34	6	28		10
	4GCD6	96	0	89	7	43
	4GCD8	96	2	90	4	27

Rejection grade[1]	Culture	[2]	[3]	[3]	[4]	[5]
2	5GCD2	44	28	9	4*	1
	5GCD4	31	6	20	3*	9
	5GCD6	96	9	68	14*	70
	5GCD8	96	2	42	52	90
1	6GCD2	4	2	2	0·	0
	6GCD4	11	4	6	1	0
	6GCD6	25	1	23	1	0
	6GCD8	4	3	1	0	0
1	9GCD2	0				
	9GCD4	3	nt	nt	nt	0
	9GCD6	16	nt	nt	nt	0
	9GCD8	42	nt	nt	nt	0

Characteristics of the mini-bulk cultures established from seven EMB of PATA at four different propagation times. At all time points 96 well cultures were started. [1] Rejection grade according to the Billingham criteria. [2] Number of wells with lymphoid cells. [3] Number of wells in which 90% or more of the TCR-αβ T cells were of the CD4 subpopulation, or of the CD8 subset. [4] Number of wells in which none of the two subsets enclose more than 89% of the αβ T cells. [5] Number of wells with T cells cytotoxic for donor B-LCL. * In the other wells, NK cells or TCR-γδ T cells were the predominant (90% or more) lymphoid cells.

Table 6.3A. PATC

HIST[1]	EMB minibulk	Growth	Phenotype			Donor specific CML
		#2	WT31CD4+ #3	WT31CD8+ #3	WT31CD4+ WT31CD8+ #4	#5
0	1GCD2	59	28	22	7*	2
	1GCD4	6	3	3		0
	1GCD6	0				
	1GCD8	7	7			
0	2GCD2	5	4	1		0
	2GCD4	0				
	2GCD6	0				
	2GCD8	0				
2	3GCD2	73	38	23	11*	3
	3GCD4	31	18	10	2*	NT
	3GCD6	96	3	34	59	81
	3GCD8	96	11	16	69	84

0					
4GCD2	47	22	20	5	0
4GCD4	16	13	3		2
4GCD6	23	8	14	1	1
4GCD8	96	75	6	15	6
1					
5GCD2	91	43	19	29	36
5GCD4	56	22	22	10*	19
5GCD6	96	24	43	24*	23
5GCD8	91	61	5	23*	14
1					
6GCD2	9	5	4		0
6GCD4	10	9	1		0
6GCD6	96	39	20	36*	70
6GCD8	96	48	20	27*	63
1					
7GCD2	43	19	8	17	18
7GCD4	50	37	11	11	10
7GCD6	94	45	4	45	90
7GCD8	94	46	0	46	84

Table 6.3B. PATC

HIST[1]	EMB minibulk	Growth	Phenotype			Donor specific CML
		#[2]	WT31CD4+ #[3]	WT31CD8+ #[3]	WT31CD4+ WT31CD8+[4]	#[5]
1	8GCD2	96	58	6	32	9
	8GCD4	21	14	6	1	5
	8GCD6	65	34	18	6	27
	8GCD8	93	4	77	13*	52
1	9GCD2	48	19	18	1*	1
	9GCD4	14	4	8	1	0
	9GCD6	24	4	20		2
	9GD8	96	1	95		3
1	10GCD2	72	26	35	11	3
	10GCD4	78	48	15	15	2
	10GCD6	96	43	1	52	95
	10GCD8	96	7	3	86	79

Culture	[1]	[2]	[3]	[4]	[5]	[*]
11GCD2	1	0					1
11GCD4		3	2				1
11GCD6		13	13				0
11GCD8		26	22			1	0
12GCD2	0	91	17	33	41	11
12GCD4		92	32	28	32	3
12GCD6		92	17	31	44	25
12GCD8		96	9	62	25	6

Characteristics of the mini-bulk cultures established from 12 EMB of PATC at four different propagation times. At all time points 96 well cultures were started. [1]Rejection grade according to the Billingham criteria. [2]Number of wells with lymphoid cells. [3]Number of wells in which 90% or more of the TCR-αβ T cells were of the CD4 subpopulation, or of the CD8 subset. [4]Number of wells in which none of the two subsets enclose more than 89% of the αβ T cells. [5]Number of wells with T cells cytotoxic for donor B-LCL. [*]In the other wells, NK cells or TCR γδ T cells were the predominant (90% or more) lymphoid cells.

The contents on T subsets of the cultures was very diverse. For PATA most mini-bulks of EMB4 and 5 contained predominantly CD8 T cells. From the mini cultures GCD2 of both EMB 4 and 5, approximately 50% contained predominantly CD4 T cells, whereas GCD8 of the rejection EMB most mini-bulks contained nearly equal amounts of CD8 and CD4 T cells. For PATC in only four timepoints (8GCD8, 9GCD6, 9GCD8 and 12GCD8) mini bulk cultures in which CD8 positive T cells predominated, formed the majority of the cultures established. At 8 timepoints (3GCD2, 3GCD4, 4GCD8, 5GCD8, 7GCD4, 8GCD2, 8GCD4 and 10GCD4) cultures with predominantly CD4 cells formed the majority. For the other culture timepoint of this patient all three

---

Table 6.4. Histological evaluation, phenotypic characterization by surface staining and cytolytic capability of the EMB derived bulk T-cell lines

	EMB	days[1]	hist.[2]	imm.[3]	CD4	CD8	cyt.[4]
PATA	1	8	1		3	97	-
	2	15	1		5	95	-
	4	29	1		10	90	+
	5	36	2	RATG	14	86	+
	6	58	1		11	89	-
	9	129	1		1	99	-
PATB	1	91	2	predn.	nd[5]	19	+
	2	137	2	predn.	nd	59	+
	3	147	2	RATG	nd	91	+
	4	210	2	predn.	nd	58	+
PATC	1	7	0		60	40	
	2	15	0		81	10	-
	3	22	2	RATG	80	20	+
	4	42	0		89	10	-
	5	49	1		71	29	+
	6	57	1		81	18	+
	7	70	1		8	91	+
	8	87	1		0	99	+
	9	112	1		0	99	-
	10	140	1		95	5	+
	11	192	1		92	8	-
	12	232	0		16	84	+

[1]days posttransplantation [2]histological evaluation according to the Billingham criteria [3]immunosuppressive treatment of rejection (RATG: Rabbit anti-thymocyte globulin, predn.:methylprednisolon) [4]cytolytic activity as defined by cell mediated lymphocytotoxicity against a panel of EBV transformed B-cell lines sharing at least one of the MHC-class I mismatches with the heart transplant donor [5]not determined.

possibilities: predominantly CD4 cells; predominantly CD8 cells and mixed cultures were nearly equally represented. No clear pattern could be extracted from these data.

In the bulk cultures all cells expressed the CD3-protein ensemble and the $\alpha\beta$ T cell receptor. All T cell lines derived from PATA were predominantly CD4$^-$CD8$^+$. In contrast, the T cell lines propagated from the EMB of PATB and PATC exhibited a different phenotype (see Table 6.4). In PATB and PATC a number of cell lines exhibited a mixed CD4$^+$CD8$^-$ and CD4$^-$CD8$^+$ character, whereas both in PATB and PATC cell lines were established in which CD4$^+$CD8$^-$ T cells predominated. Independent of the outcome of the histological evaluation, the established bulk T cell lines exhibited cytolytic activity against donor or HLA matched B-LCL. Bulk T cell lines established from grade 1 biopsies did not always manifest cytolytic activity, while bulk T cell lines established from grade 2 biopsies were always cytolytic against donor and/or HLA matched B-LCL. From three T cell lines derived from grade 2 biopsies T cell clones were established. The cytolytic T cell lines and T cell clones of the patients were further investigated against a panel of allogenic EBV-transformed B cell lines (not shown). Various specificities could be determined. Several clones of PATA.5 shared reactivity against the HLA-A29 antigen, while clones of PATB.3 showed specific reactivity against the HLA-B60, HLA-B40, HLA-B62 and HLA-A11 antigens. Four out of six of the seeded T cell lines established from patient PATC (PATC.6, PATC.7, PATC.9 and PATC.12) only lysed B-LCL that shared the HLA-B62 antigen. Inhibition experiments with monoclonal antibodies directed against HLA class I and CD3 could inhibit the cytolytic activity of the HLA-A29 specific clones, confirming the TCR/CD3 mediated reactivity against this class-I antigen. Anti-CD8 did not inhibit the lysis which is indicative for the high affinity of the T cell receptor for this allo-MHC/peptide complex.

6.3.2 TCR V-region Analysis of Allo-MHC Class I Specific CTL Lines

Using a number of the currently available monoclonal antibodies directed against defined TCR V gene segments, we could only detect a few of the TCR V family gene segments in the T cell lines propagated from the graft-infiltrating T lymphocytes when compared to T cell cultures generated from samples of peripheral blood mononuclear cells of patient PATA (PBMCPATA.6, Table 6.5). In some of the T cell lines derived from different biopsies a predominance of defined T cell receptor V regions was noted (for example, see patient PATA which expressed almost exclusively the TCRBV6S7 gene segment in biopsy derived T cell line PATA.6). Similarly patient PATB expressed relative high levels of TCRBV8S1 in the T cell line PATB.2 and of TCRBV2S1 and TCRBV5S2/3 gene segments in the T cell line PATB.4 (Table 6.5).

Table 6.5. Cell surface expression of TCR V gene segments as determined by FACS analysis of some of three of the T cell lines of PATA, the PBMC derived T cell line of PATA and all T cell lines of PATB

cell line	Percentage of stained cells													
	TCRBV												TCRAV	
	2	3	5.1	5.2/3	5.3	6.7	8.1	8	12	13	17	19	2	12
PATA.4	nd	nd	nd	8	0	0	nd	0	0	nd	nd	nd	0	nd
PATA.5	nd	nd	nd	0	0	0	nd	13	0	nd	nd	nd	0	nd
PATA.6	nd	nd	nd	0	0	88	nd	0	0	nd	nd	nd	0	nd
PBMCPATA.6	nd	nd	nd	5	1	2	nd	5	2	nd	nd	nd	4	nd
PATB.1	1	0	0	0	0	nd	1	1	1	0	0	0	8	3
PATB.2	18	0	0	6	0	nd	34	14	1	0	0	0	0	3
PATB.3	0	0	9	0	1	nd	0	0	2	1	0	0	3	0
PATB.4	30	0	0	30	27	nd	0	0	1	1	1	1	3	0

Table 6.6. TCRBV gene segment usage of T-lymphocyte cell lines derived from EMBs taken from three different heart transplant patients and of two PBMC derived T cell lines of PATA; PBMCPATA.0 was taken before transplantation, PBMCPATA.6 was taken at the same time as biopsy PATA.6

T cell line	1	2	3	4	5	6	7	8	9	10	11	12	13	14	15	16	17	18	19	20	21	22	23	24
PATA.1							+						nd				+	+			nd	nd	nd	nd
PATA.2													nd	+				+			nd	nd	nd	nd
PATA.4	+		+		+	+	+	+	+				nd	+			+	+		+	nd	nd	nd	nd
PATA.5	+		+			+	+	+					nd	+			+	+	+	+	nd	nd	nd	nd
PATA.6						+		+					nd					+			nd	nd	nd	nd
PATA.9							+		+	+		+	nd	+			+	+	+		nd	nd	nd	nd
PBMCPATA.0	+	+	+	+	+	+	+	+	+	+	+	+	nd	+	+	+	+	+	+	+	nd	nd	nd	nd
PBMCPATA.6	+	+	+	+	+	+	+	+	+	+	+	+	nd	+	+	+	+	+	+	+	nd	nd	nd	nd
PATB.1	+	+	+	+	+	+	+	+	+		+		+	+			+	+	+		+	+		
PATB.2	+	+	+		+	+	+	+	+				+	+	+			+	+		+	+	+	
PATB.3				+	+						+		+	+										
PATB.4		+			+	+		+					+		+				+		+			
PATC.3					+		+	+						+					+					
PATC.6			+	+										+										
PATC.7			+	+									+	+				+			+			
PATC.8				+	+																			
PATC.10		+		+					+									+	+					
PATC.12	+					+						+												

Since these types of analysis do not allow the description of the complete T cell receptor gene repertoire we have expanded these studies and have analyzed T cell receptor V-gene use in the various endomycard biopsy derived T cell lines at the transcriptional level by RT-PCR. As can be seen from Table 6.6 these analyses showed that each graft-infiltrating T cell line exhibited a different pattern of TCRBV gene usage. In general, the number of TCRBV gene segments which were used by the T cell lines, propagated from endomyocardium infiltrating T-lymphocytes were restricted when compared to the T cell lines derived from PBMC. In the PBMC derived T cell lines all TCRBV genes could be detected. Despite different patterns of TCR V gene usage in the different graft-infiltrating T lymphocyte cell lines there is an apparent sharing of defined TCR V gene families by some of the T cell lines tested in the individual patients. This is exemplified by the sharing of TCRBV 6, 7, 14, 17 and 18 in the different graft infiltrating T lymphocyte cell lines of patient PATA. Similarly, the various T cell lines of patient PATC, which were selected on basis of their cytolytic activity, shared the TCRBV4 gene family in five out of six T cell lines. It should be noted that each patient exhibited an individual specific pattern of the TCRBV gene expression and sharing of these TCR V-regions among the various graft-infiltrating T lymphocyte cell lines. Subsequent analysis to the level of TCRAV and TCRBV expression in patient PATA, as defined by densitometry, showed that some of the TCRBV as well as the TCRAV gene segments including the shared TCR V genes were used at high frequencies in the various T cell lines when compared with the other TCR V genes used by the same T cell lines (see Figs. 6.1 and 6.2). In general, the various TCRAV and TCRBV genes were expressed at different levels in the T cell lines propagated from graft-infiltrating T-lymphocytes.

In case of PATA an expansion of the TCRAV and TCRBV repertoires was noted in time, which seems to be associated with the rejection crises as determined by the Billingham criteria. Treatment with anti thymocyte globulin (RATG) resulted in a clear declination in the spectrum of TCR V gene families used in patient PATA (see Figs. 6.1 and 6.2).

The T cell lines derived from patient PATB, which were all derived from grade 2 biopsies, exhibited in general a more polyclonal character as deduced from the number of TCRBV families which could be detected by RT-PCR in the T-cell lines. However, not all T cell lines derived from grade 2 biopsies exhibit this polyclonal character. In PATC we observed a paucity in the number of TCRBV gene families employed by grade 2 derived T cells in PATC.3.

6.3.3 STRUCTURE OF THE TCR α AND β CHAINS OF T CELL CLONES SPECIFIC FOR ALLO-MHC

To investigate the structure of the TCR α and β chains used by allo-specific T cell clones in more detail, we have analyzed 26 T cell

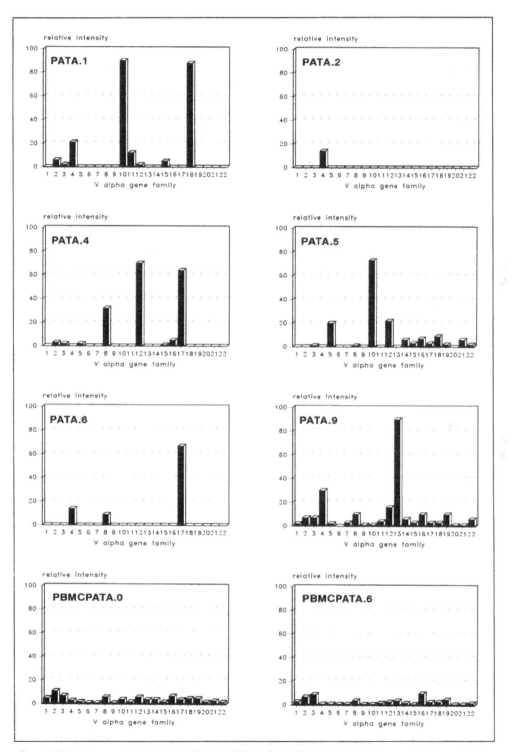

Fig. 6.1 TCRAV gene segment usage of GITL cell lines derived from six EMBs of PATA and two T cell lines generated from PBMC taken before transplantation (PBMCPATA.0) and at time of EMB PATA.6 (PBMCPATA6). Reprinted with minor modifications from Datema et al. Transplantation 1994; 57:119-26

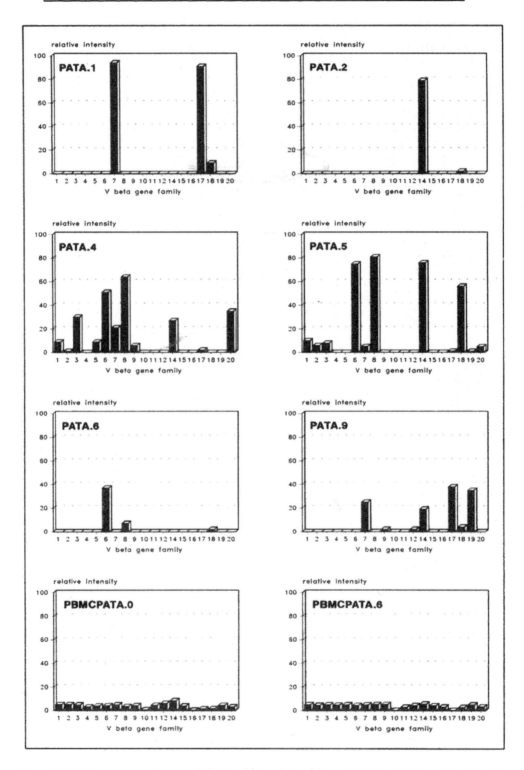

Fig. 6.2 TCRBV gene segment usage of GITL cell lines derived from six EMBs of PATA and two T cell lines generated from PBMC taken before transplantation (PBMCPATA.0) and at time of EMB PATA.6 (PBMCPATA6). Reprinted with minor modifications from Datema et al. Transplantation 1994; 57: 1119-26.

clones which were derived from cytolytic graft-infiltrating T lymphocyte cell lines from two different cardiac transplant patients. As can been seen from Table 6.7, not all clones manifested cytolytic activity against donor B-LCL. It is to note that the majority of these non-cytolytic clones were CD4⁺CD8⁻, whereas all cytolytic T cell clones exhibited the CD4⁻CD8⁺ phenotype with the exception of two clones established from PATB.3 which expressed simultaneously both the CD4 and CD8 antigens.

Panel analyses, to determine the HLA specificity of these various cytolytic T cell clones derived from graft-infiltrating T-lymphocytes, showed that in PATA the cytolytic clones recognized HLA-A29, whereas the cytolytic clones from PATB.3 and PATB.4 recognized the HLA-B62, B40 and HLA-B62, B40, B60 and A11 respectively. The analysis of the TCRAV and TCRBV gene family usage of the various cytolytic clones revealed an heterogeneous usage pattern as tabulated in Table 6.7. The HLA-A29 restricted cytolytic T cell clones from PATA expressed the TCRAV10 and TCRBV20 genes. Depending on the alloantigen that was recognized, the various T cell clones employed different combinations of TCRAV and TCRBV genes within each patient. In patient PATB, the cytolytic T cell clones, that were established from two different grade 2 biopsy T cell lines that showed reactivity against the same HLA-B62 or HLA-B40 antigen used different TCRAV/ TCRBV gene family combinations. Furthermore, the HLA-B62 and HLA-B60 specific T cell clones that were derived from T cell line

Table 6.7. Specificity, phenotype and TCRAV and TCRBV gene segment usage of T cell clones generated from three EMB derived T cell lines

Patient	spec.[1]	no.[2]	CD	TCRAV	TCRBV
PATA.5	A29	4	8	10	20
	nc[3]	6	8	5	6
	nc	2	4	21	14
	nc	1	4	4	6
PATB.3	B62	1	8	2	4
	B40[4]	2	8/4[5]	6	14
	nc	2	4	14,16	12
PATB.4	B62	2	8	6	5
	B40	2	8	11	2
	B60	1	8	7	5
	A11	1	8	16	21
	nc	2	4	20	13

[1]HLA specificity as determined by panel analysis. [2]no. of clones analyzed. [3]no cytotoxicity. [4]T cell clones recognized both the HLA-B40 splits (HLA-B60 and HLA-B61). [5]The double positive nature of these clones was confirmed by staining with anti CD8 β-chain monoclonal.

PATB.4 both used the TCRBV5S3 gene segment. Comparison of the TCRV gene family analysis as presented in Tables 6.6 and 6.7 shows that the TCR V genes used in the allo-specific cytolytic T cell clones were readily detectable in the endomyocard derived cell lines.

To gain more insight in the structural aspects of the TCRs used in allo-specific recognition, we have determined the nucleotide sequence of the TCR V regions and analyzed the deduced amino acid composition including the CDR3 region of both the α and β chain of TCRs used by the different cytolytic T cell clones and non-cytolytic T cell clones. As can been seen from Table 6.8, the TCR β chain CDR3 region amino acid composition of different T-cell clones, including T cell clones with the same HLA class-I specificity, showed a diverse usage pattern of amino acids. Similarly, analysis of the TCR β chain CDR3 regions of T-cell clones of PATA and PATB, both cytolytic and non-cytolytic also revealed a heterogeneous usage pattern of amino acids in the CDR3 region. As can been seen from Table 6.8, the CDR3 region of the HLA-B40 restricted cytolytic T cell clones derived from PATB.3 and PATB.4 also differed.

The question, whether the cytolytic T cell clones established from grade 2 biopsies could also be detected in previously taken biopsies, was addressed in more detail in PATA. The presence of the CDR3 region of the TCRBV20S1 gene segment, used by the HLA-A29 specific T-cell clones derived from PATA.5, in the TCRBV20 PCR product of cell line PATA.4, was examined taking advantage of an oligonucleotide specific for the CDR3 region. These hybridization analysis revealed that the cytolytic CDR3 regions were not present in the cell line from PATA.4 (see Datema et al.[36]). Also, we were not able to detect these sequences among peripheral blood mononuclear cells, taken at the same time as PATA.5, indicating that these effector T cells were present at extremely low concentrations in the periphery. The occurrence of identical V, N-D-N and J regions revealed that a number of T cell clones derived from the graft infiltrating T-lymphocyte cell lines were derived from the same progenitor. Whether this progenitor T cell clone was already amplified in the endomycard biopsy or whether this progenitor as a consequence of previous activation in the endomyocard was preferentially amplified during the generation of the graft-infiltrating T lymphocyte cell line remains to be investigated.

6.4 DISCUSSION

Graft-infiltrating T lymphocytes, which were polyclonally propagated from sequentially taken EMB from heart transplant patients showed a consistent propagation pattern. In general, most T cell cultures established in the first 4 days of culture did not recognize donor specific MHC/peptide complexes as determined by cytotoxicity assays. Those cytotoxic T cells however, were abundantly present in the majority of the later established cultures. Most T cells propagated in the first 4 days

QUESTIONNAIRE

Receive a FREE BOOK of your choice

Please help us out—Just answer the questions below, then select the book of your choice from the list on the back and return this card.

R.G. Landes Company publishes five book series: *Medical Intelligence Unit, Molecular Biology Intelligence Unit, Neuroscience Intelligence Unit, Tissue Engineering Intelligence Unit* and *Biotechnology Intelligence Unit.* We also publish comprehensive, shorter than book-length reports on well-circumscribed topics in molecular biology and medicine. The authors of our books and reports are acknowledged leaders in their fields and the topics are unique. Almost without exception, there are no other comprehensive publications on these topics.

Our goal is to publish material in important and rapidly changing areas of bioscience for sophisticated scientists. To achieve this goal, we have accelerated our publishing program to conform to the fast pace in which information grows in bioscience. Most of our books and reports are published within 90 to 120 days of receipt of the manuscript.

Please circle your response to the questions below.

1. We would like to sell our *books* to scientists and students at a deep discount. But we can only do this as part of a prepaid subscription program. The retail price range for our books is $59-$99. Would you pay $196 to select four *books* per year from any of our Intelligence Units–$49 per book–as part of a prepaid program?

    Yes   **No**

2. We would like to sell our *reports* to scientists and students at a deep discount. But we can only do this as part of a prepaid subscription program. The retail price range for our reports is $39-$59. Would you pay $145 to select five *reports* per year–$29 per report–as part of a prepaid program?

    Yes   **No**

3. Would you pay $39–the retail price range of our books is $59-$99–to receive any single book in our Intelligence Units if it is spiral bound, but in every other way identical to the more expensive hardcover version?

    Yes   **No**

To receive your free book, please fill out the shipping information below, select your free book choice from the list on the back of this survey and mail this card to:

R.G. Landes Company, 909 S. Pine Street, Georgetown, Texas 78626 U.S.A.

Your Name _____

Address _____

City _____ State/Province: _____

Country: _____ Postal Code: _____

My computer type is Macintosh _____ ; IBM-compatible _____ ; Other _____

Do you own _____ or plan to purchase _____ a CD-ROM drive?

Available Free Titles

Please check three titles in order of preference.
Your request will be filled based on availability. Thank you.

☐ Water Channels
Alan Verkman,
University of California-San Francisco

☐ The Na,K-ATPase:
Structure-Function Relationship
J.-D. Horisberger, University of Lausanne

☐ Intrathymic Development of T Cells
J. Nikolic-Zugic,
Memorial Sloan-Kettering Cancer Center

☐ Cyclic GMP
Thomas Lincoln, University of Alabama

☐ Primordial VRM System and the Evolution
of Vertebrate Immunity
John Stewart, Institut Pasteur-Paris

☐ Thyroid Hormone Regulation
of Gene Expression
Graham R. Williams, University of Birmingham

☐ Mechanisms of Immunological Self Tolerance
Guido Kroemer, CNRS Génétique Moléculaire et
Biologie du Développement-Villejuif

☐ The Costimulatory Pathway
for T Cell Responses
Yang Liu, New York University

☐ Molecular Genetics of Drosophila Oogenesis
Paul F. Lasko, McGill University

☐ Mechanism of Steroid Hormone Regulation
of Gene Transcription
M.-J. Tsai & Bert W. O'Malley, Baylor University

☐ Liver Gene Expression
François Tronche & Moshe Yaniv,
Institut Pasteur-Paris

☐ RNA Polymerase III Transcription
R.J. White, University of Cambridge

☐ src Family of Tyrosine Kinases in Leukocytes
Tomas Mustelin, La Jolla Institute

☐ MHC Antigens and NK Cells
Rafael Solana & Jose Peña,
University of Córdoba

☐ Kinetic Modeling of Gene Expression
James L. Hargrove, University of Georgia

☐ PCR and the Analysis of the T Cell Receptor
Repertoire
Jorge Oksenberg, Michael Panzara & Lawrence
Steinman, Stanford University

☐ Myointimal Hyperplasia
Philip Dobrin, Loyola University

☐ Transgenic Mice as an In Vivo Model
of Self-Reactivity
David Ferrick & Lisa DiMolfetto-Landon,
University of California-Davis and Pamela Ohashi,
Ontario Cancer Institute

☐ Cytogenetics of Bone and Soft Tissue Tumors
Avery A. Sandberg, Genetrix & Julia A. Bridge ,
University of Nebraska

☐ The Th1-Th2 Paradigm and Transplantation
Robin Lowry, Emory University

☐ Phagocyte Production and Function Following
Thermal Injury
Verlyn Peterson & Daniel R. Ambruso,
University of Colorado

☐ Human T Lymphocyte Activation Deficiencies
José Regueiro, Carlos Rodríguez-Gallego
and Antonio Arnaiz-Villena,
Hospital 12 de Octubre-Madrid

☐ Monoclonal Antibody in Detection and
Treatment of Colon Cancer
Edward W. Martin, Jr., Ohio State University

☐ Enteric Physiology of the Transplanted Intestine
Michael Sarr & Nadey S. Hakim, Mayo Clinic

☐ Artificial Chordae in Mitral Valve Surgery
Claudio Zussa, S. Maria dei Battuti Hospital-Treviso

☐ Injury and Tumor Implantation
Satya Murthy & Edward Scanlon,
Northwestern University

☐ Support of the Acutely Failing Liver
A.A. Demetriou, Cedars-Sinai

☐ Reactive Metabolites of Oxygen and Nitrogen
in Biology and Medicine
Matthew Grisham, Louisiana State-Shreveport

☐ Biology of Lung Cancer
Adi Gazdar & Paul Carbone,
Southwestern Medical Center

☐ Quantitative Measurement
of Venous Incompetence
Paul S. van Bemmelen, Southern Illinois University
and John J. Bergan, Scripps Memorial Hospital

☐ Adhesion Molecules in Organ Transplants
Gustav Steinhoff, University of Kiel

☐ Purging in Bone Marrow Transplantation
Subhash C. Gulati,
Memorial Sloan-Kettering Cancer Center

☐ Trauma 2000: Strategies for the New Millennium
David J. Dries & Richard L. Gamelli,
Loyola University

Table 6.8 V,D,J and C region determination by sequence analysis of T cell clones

clone	spec.	V		N	J	V		NDN	J
PATA.5	A29	10	CA	AD	GGS 42	20	CAWS	VGPA	YGY 1.2
	nc					6.4	CASSL	DRP	QYF 2.5
PATA.4	nc					6.6/7	CASSL	LPL	NEQ 2.1
PATB.4	B62	6	CA	MRRT	NDY 20	5.3	CASS	IRQY	TGE 2.2
	B60	7	CA	RA	TTD 24	5.3	CASS	PGQGAV	DTQ 2.3
	B40	11	CAV	KG	YGQ 26	2	CSAR	DPSGR	SYE 2.7
	A11	16	CAVR	DLVD	SGY 41	21	nd		
	nc	13	CL	VG	YGG 42	13	S	PTGSG	KTV 1.3
PATB.3	B62	2	nd			4.1	CSV	DSAITT	FG 1.2
	B40	6	CA	MRRD	FKK 21	14	CASSL	SGAI	NQP 1.5
	nc	14	CA	YRSVD	SGT 40	12.2	CAIS	TGTRPL	ETQ 2.5
		16	CAVR	DA	GNQ 49				

of culture may represent cytotoxic T cell precursors (CTLp) with donor specificity or with specificity for irrelevant antigens. In a previous study we have demonstrated that CTLp with donor specificity were present at high frequency in T cell cultures propagated from EMB, even when they were cultured only in the presence of IL-2 and autologous feeder cells.[37] Also CTLp without specificity for donor HLA antigens were found to be present.[38,39] Those CTLp may reflect PBMC passing the grafts capillary system at the moment the EMB was taken or may be attracted "aspecific" to the graft as a result of the donor directed immune response as shown by Orosz et al.[40] Since CTLp are not activated they are not directly engaged in the binding of donor MHC/peptide complexes in the EMB and as a consequence could leave the biopsy earlier during culture when compared to the activated donor directed CTL which is engaged in active binding to their target structure. These CTL leave the EMB when it starts to disintegrate due to in vitro cultures conditions which were not optimal for endothelial cells, myocytes and connective tissue. Biopsy 5 of PATC was the only exception, from this biopsy the day 2 culture gave most cytotoxic mini bulks. Since this was the biopsy following the control biopsy for rejection treatment, in which only a few mini bulk cultures showed cytolytic activity against donor cells, we interpreted this as activated donor directed CTL, present in the capillary system, that repopulated the graft. In the following biopsies the donor directed CTL were again predominantly present in the minibulk cultures propagated at 6 days or later. That those CTL did not cause rejection might be because they have low avidity for donor antigens, were more sensitive for cyclosporin A (CsA), and were present at a lower frequency. In other studies, we have shown that CTL present in the graft during or before rejection had high avidity for donor antigens and were resistant for CsA, whereas CTL in EMB without rejection had low avidity, were more sensitive to CsA and were present at lower frequencies.[37,38,41]

Both the TCRAV and TCRBV repertoires in the various cytotoxic T cell lines were extensive though smaller than the peripheral TCRAV and TCRBV repertoires on the basis of the numbers of expressed TCR V-gene families. Subsequent establishment of allo-specific cytolytic T-cell clones revealed that various donor encoded HLA specificities could be detected among these clones. The nucleotide sequence analysis of the TCRAV and TCRBV regions of these cytolytic T cell clones established from the same T cell line has shown that a number of cytolytic T cell clones displaying shared specificities expressed identical TCRAV and TCRBV regions. This suggests that these T cell clones were all derived from the same progenitor. However, cytolytic T cell clones, established from different T cell lines but sharing HLA-specificity, expressed different TCRAV and TCRBV regions.

Propagation and sequencing of T cell clones isolated from GITL cell line PATA.5 showed that all T cell clones that recognized donor

B-LCL in a MHC restricted fashion were using identical TCR A αvδ B V-regions. The TCRBV20 gene product used by these clones is detectable in cell line PATA.5 albeit at a relative low frequency. This in contrast to the other TCR V-genes that were detected in PATA.4 which exhibited relative higher expression patterns. However, T cell clones employing TCRBV6S4 genes did not manifest donor specific reactivity. Furthermore, using a CDR3 region specific oligonucleotide we were able to demonstrate that this sequence could only be detected in PATA.5 and not in PATA.4 showing that among the relatively more abundant TCRBV20, as detected by PCR, the cytotoxic T cell clone progenitor of PATA.5 was not present.

However, it is possible that T cells which initiate the rejection episode are detected in GITL cell line PATA.4 and may be represented by the T cells that employ TCR V-regions that differ from the TCR V regions employed by the effector T cells that are responsible for the tissue damage. This is supported by the observation made in PATB. In PATB (PATB.3 and PATB.4) the cytolytic T cell clones with shared specificities displayed usage of different TCRAV and TCRBV regions. These clones were derived from cytotoxic T cell lines established from sequentially taken grade 2 rejection biopsies, suggesting that indeed the effector functions can be performed by different T cell clones. Alternatively, this observation could also imply that T cells that are mediating tissue damage are unique at a certain timepoint following transplantation and as a consequence, these effector T cells might not be identifiable at other timepoints after transplantation.

The function of the other T cells that use TCR V-genes like BV6, 8 and 14, which are predominant in the GITL cell line PATA.4 and PATA.5 for instance, remains to be investigated further. These αβ TCR might recognize the HLA alloantigens only in combination with endothelial or endomyocard specific peptides which are also possible targets for an alloreactive response causing tissue destruction.

T cell clones established from patient PATB (PATB.3 and PATB.4) showed identical HLA class I specificities (HLA-B62 and HLA-B40), despite the fact that they used different TCRAV/TCRBV gene combinations.

In the biopsies taken at earlier time points following transplantation of PATA only a limited number of TCRAV and TCRBV genes could been detected. This was seen particular in GITL cell lines derived from grade 1 EMB that exhibited no cytolytic activity in vitro. In GITL cell lines derived from rejection EMB that exhibited specific cytolytic activity in vitro, the TCR V-gene repertoire was more extensive. However, when compared to T cell lines derived from purified samples of PBMC, the TCR V-gene repertoire in these EMB was limited. Since the cultures used for TCRAV and TCRBV repertoire analysis from PATC were day 6 or day 8 mini-bulk cultures the more restricted pattern in TCR V gene usage might represent more accurately the donor directed T cells. From PATA and PATB bulk cultures were used for these analysis in which beside donor directed T cells also T cells might be present with irrelevant specificities as discussed before. This may lead to a more broad type of TCRVB repertoire.

An other explanation for the apparent utilization of only a limited number of TCR V-genes by GITL cell lines might be that the starting number of T cells present in the original biopsy is below the amount of T cells that is needed to describe a complete T cell repertoire allowing the detecting of all TCR V-genes. Wyngaard et al.[42] showed that the maximal number of CD3+ cells detected in grade 1 biopsies by immunolabeling did not exceed 200 cells/mm². However, the observed sharing of certain TCR V family genes by some of the GITL cell lines supports the idea of a restricted usage of TCR V-gene segments by GITL. Also, the apparent restriction in the number of T cell receptor V-gene families in the T cell lines established from endomyocard infiltrating T cells might be the results of selection in vivo for allo-specific T cell clones. In a study by Hall et al.[43] it was shown that the T cell receptor repertoire of unstimulated peripheral blood lymphocytes became compressed in a long-term mixed lymphocyte reaction as a consequence of repeated allogeneic stimulation in vitro. These observations suggests that the T cell receptor repertoire of allo specific T cell clones could be restricted in nature. The presence of a relative extensive TCR V gene repertoire both in PATA.4, PATA.5, PATB.1 and PATB.2 could be the result of attraction to the site of inflammation of non-specific T cells, by events such as increased production of cytokines and growth factors by graft infiltrating regulating T cells[44] or, through presentation of novel antigenic peptides as a consequence of tissue damage by cytotoxic T cells.

In conclusion, our study indicates that in GITL propagated from biopsies, taken at different time points from three cardiac transplant patients, in general fewer TCR V gene families could be detected as found among PBMC. Some of these TCR V genes were shared by different GITL cell lines which is indicative of a restricted usage of TCR V genes by GITL, However, T cells that were able to lyse donor B-LCL in a MHC class I restricted fashion, as determined by T cell cloning and sequence analysis, were only detected in grade 2 biopsies taken at the time of rejection. No evidence was found for the presence of identical cytolytic T cells in multiple biopsies taken at different time points, suggesting that T cells exhibiting donor specific cytolytic activity have been recently recruited towards the endomyocard.

ACKNOWLEDGMENTS

This research was supported by the Eurotransplant Foundation, The Netherlands Heart Foundation and the J.A. Cohen Institute for Radiopathology and Radiation Protection (IRS).

REFERENCES

1. Billingham ME. Diagnosis of cardiac rejection by endomyocardial biopsy. Heart Transplantation 1982; 1:25-30.
2. Lechler RI, Lombardi G, Batchelor JR et al. The molecular basis of alloreactivity. Immunol Today 1990; 11:83-8.
3. Eckels DD, Gorski J, Rothbard J et al. Peptide-mediated modulation of T-cell alloregcognition. Proc Natl Acad Sci 1988; 85:8191-5.
4. McWhinnie DL, Thompson JF, Taylor HM et al. Morphometric analysis of cellular infiltration assessed by monoclonal antibody labeling in sequential human renal allograft biopsies. Transplantation 1986; 42:352-8.
5. Saidman SL, Demitris AJ, Zeevi A et al. Propagation of lymphocytes infiltrating human liver allografts. Transplantation 1990; 49:107-12.
6. Kaufmann CL, Zeevi A, Kormos RL et al. Propagation of infiltrating lymphocytes and graft coronary disease in cardiac transplant recipients. Hum Immunol 1990; 28:228-36.
7. Zeevi A, Fung J, Zerbe TR et al. Allospecificity of activated T cells grown from endomyocardial biopsies from heart transplant patients. Transplantation 1986; 41:620-26.
8. Mayer TG, Fuller AA, Fuller TC et al. Characterization of in vivo-activated allospecific T-lymphocytes propagated from human renal allograft biopsies undergoing rejection. J Immunol 1985; 134:258-64.
9. Micelli MC, Todd TS and Finn OJ. Human allograft-derived T-cell lines: Donor class I- and class II- directed cytotoxicity and repertoire stability in sequential biopsies. Hum Immunol 1988; 22:185-98.
10. Ouwehand AJ, Vaessen LMB, Baan CC et al. Alloreactive lymphoid infiltrates in human heart transplants. Hum Immunol 1991; 30:50-9.
11. Trentin L, Zambello R, Faggian G et al. Phenotypic and functional characterization of cytotoxic cells derived from endomyocardial biopsies in human cardiac allografts. Cell Immunol 1992; 141:332-41.
12. Davis MM and Bjorkman PJ. T-cell antigen receptor genes and T-cell recognition. Nature 1988; 334:395-402.
13. Chothia C, Boswell DR and Lesk AM. The outline structure of the T cell αβ receptor. E.M.B.O. 1988; 7:3745-55.
14. Claverie J-M, Prochnicka-Chalufour A and Bougueleret L. Implications of a Fab-like structure for the T-cell receptor. Immunol Today 1989; 10:10-3.
15. Engel I and Hedrick SM. Site-directed mutation in the VDJ junctional region of a T-cell receptor β cause changes in antigenic peptide recognition. Cell 1988; 54:473-84.
16. Sorger SB, Paterson Y, Fink PJ et al. T cell receptor junctional regions and the MHC molecule affect recognition of antigenic peptides by T cell clones. J Immunol 1990; 144:1127-35.
17. Danska JS, Livingstone AM, Paragas V et al. The presumptive CDR3 region of both T cell receptor α and β chains determine T cell specificity for myoglobin peptides. J Exp Med 1990; 172:27-33.

18. Jorgensen JL, Esser U, Fazekas de Groth B et al. Mapping T-cell receptor-peptide contacts by variant peptide immunization of single-chain transgenic. Nature 1992; 355:224-30.

19. Wucherpfennnig KW, Ota K, Endo N et al. Shared human T cell receptor Vβ usage to immunodominant regions of myelin basic protein. Science 1990; 248:1016-9.

20. Moss PAH, Moots RJ, Rosenberg WMC et al. Extensive conservation of α and β chains of the human T-cell antigen receptor recognizing HLA-A2 and influenza A matrix peptide. Proc Natl Acad Sci 1991; 88:8987-90.

21. Hansen T, Qvigstad E, Lundin KAE et al. T-cell receptor β usage by 35 different antigen-specific T-cell clones restricted by HLA-Dw4 or -Dw14.1. Hum Immunol 1992; 35:149-56.

22. Van Schooten CA, Long Ko J, van der Stoep N et al. T-cell receptor β-chain gene usage in the T-cell recognition of Mycobacterium leprae antigens in one tuberloid leprosy patient. Proc Natl Acad Sci 1992; 89:11244-8.

23. Bowness P, Moss PHA, Rowland-Jones S et al. Conservation of T cell receptor usage by HLA-B27 restricted influenza-specific cytotoxic T lymphocytes suggests a general pattern for antigen-specific major histocompatibility complex I-restricted responses. J Immunol 1993; 23:1417-21.

24. Wang X-H, Ohmen JD, Uyemura K et al. Selection of T lymphocytes bearing limited T-cell receptor β chains in the response to a human pathogen. Proc Natl Acad Sci 1993; 90:188-92.

25. Wucherpfennig KW, Zhang J, Witek C et al. Clonal expansion and persistence of human T cells specific for a immunodominant myelin protein peptide. J Immunol 1994; 152:5581-92.

26. Rebai N and Malissen B. Structural and genetic analysis of HLA class I molecules using xenoantibodies. Tissue Antigens 1983; 22:107-117.

27. Liabeuf A, Le Borgne de Kaouel C, Kourilski FM et al. An antigenic determinant of human β₂-microglobulin masked by the association with HLA heavy chains at the cell surface: analysis using monoclonal antibodies. J Immunol 1981; 127: 1542-8.

28. Koning F, Schreuder GMT, Giphart MJ et al. A mouse monoclonal antibody detecting a DR-related MT2-like specificity: serology and biochemistry. Hum Immunol 1984; 4:221-30.

29. Tax WJM, Willems HW, Reekers PPM et al. Polymorphism in mitogenic effect of IgG1 monoclonal against T3 antigen on human T-cells. Nature 1983; 304:445-7.

30. Koning F. Identification and functional relevance of epitopes on human lymphocytes. PhD thesis Leiden University 1984.

31. Vandekerckhove BAE, Datema G, Koning F et al. Analysis of the donor-specific cytotoxic T-lymphocyte repertoire in a patient with a long term surviving allograft. J Immunol 1990; 144:1288-94.

32. Hawes GE, Struyk L and van den Elsen PJ. Differential usage of T cell receptor V gene segments in CD4⁺ and CD8⁺ subsets of T lymphocytes in monozygotic twins. J Immunol 1993; 150:2033-45.

33. Lambert M, van Eggermond MJCA, Mascart F. TCR Vα- and Vβ-gene segment use in T-cell subcultures derived from a type-III bare lymphocyte syndrome patient deficient in MHC class-II expression. Developmental Immunol 1992; 2:227-35.

34. Oksenberg JR, Stuart S, Begovich AB et al. Limited heterogenity of rearranged T-cell receptor Vα transcripts in brains of multiple sclerosis patients. Nature 1990 345:344-6.

35. Kenter MJH, Anholts JDH, Schreuder GMT et al. Unambiguous typing for the HLA-DQ TA10 and 2B3 specificities using oligonucleotide probes. Hum Immunol 1989; 24:65-73.

36. Datema G, Vaessen LMB, Daane RC et al. Functional and molecular characterization of graft-infiltrating T lymphocytes propagated from different biopsies derived from one heart transplant patient. Transplantation 1994; 57:1119-26.

37. Vaessen LMB, Baan CC, Ouwehand AJ et al. Differential avidity and cyclosporin sensitivity of committed donor-specific graft-infiltrating cytotoxic T cells and their precursors. Transplantation 1994; 57:1051-9.

38. Suiters AJ, Rose ML, Dominguez MJ et al. Selection for donor-specific cytotoxic T lymphocytes within the allografted human heart. Transplantation 1990; 49:1105-9.

39. Ouwehand AJ, Baan CC, Roelen DL et al. The detection of cytotoxic T cells with high affinity receptors for donor antigens in the transplanted heart as a prognostic factor for graft rejection. Transplantation 1993; 56:1223-9.

40. Orosz CG, Horstemeyer B, Zinn NE et al. Influence of graft implantation on the activation and redistribution of graft-reactive CTL. Transplantation 1989; 48:519-24.

41. Baan CC, Vaessen LMB, Loonen EHM et al. The effect of thymocyte globulin therapy on frequency and avidity of allo-specific committed CTL in clinical heart transplantation. Transplant Proc 1995; in press.

42. Wyngaard PLJ, Tuynman WB, Gmelig Meyling FHJ et al. Endomyocardial biopsies after heart transplantation. Transplantation 1993; 55:103-10.

43. Hall BL, Hand SL, Alter MD et al. Variables affecting the T cell receptor V repertoire heterogeneity of T cells infiltrating human renal allografts. Transplant Immunol 1993; 1:217-27.

44. Wu CJ, Lovett M, Wong-Lee J et al. V.A. Starnes, and C. Clayberger. Cytokine gene expression in rejecting cardiac allografts. Transplantation 1992; 54:326-32.

CHAPTER 7

INVOLVEMENT OF MINOR HISTOCOMPATABILITY ANTIGENS IN THE REJECTION OF AN HLA IDENTICAL RENAL TRANSPLANT FROM A LIVING RELATED DONOR

Benito A. Yard, Thomas Reterink, Jan Antony Bruijn,
Peter J. van den Elsen, Frans J. Claas, Mohamed R. Daha,
Leendert A. van Es and Fokko J. van der Woude

7. ABSTRACT

Graft-infiltrating T-lymphocytes (GITL) were isolated from two successive biopsies of a patient who had received an HLA-identical kidney from his brother. Both T-cell lines were highly cytotoxic against cultured proximal tubular epithelial cells (PTEC) and PHA stimulated peripheral blood lymphocytes (PBL), both of donor origin. In addition paired samples of PBL isolated at the time of the second rejection and cultured in a similar fashion as GITL displayed cytotoxicity against PTEC, although to a lesser extent. Cytotoxicity was not due to LAK activity since HLA typed target cells were specifically lysed. By using PBL from several members of the patient's family as target it was demonstrated that cytotoxicity was related to the haplotype HLA-A25, B18, CW7. Susceptibility to lysis was inherited independently from the HLA haplotypes as would be expected of minor histocompatibility antigens (mH). Using a panel of HLA typed PBL not related to the patient, a single HLA specificity could not be demonstrated.

The Human T-Cell Receptor Repertoire and Transplantation, edited by Peter J. van den Elsen. © 1995 R.G. Landes Company.

Cytotoxicity was T cell mediated and MHC class I restricted as could be shown by inhibition experiments. Adhesion between GITL and PTEC was almost completely dependent on the LFA-1/ICAM-1 adhesion pathway. The diversity of the T-cell receptor repertoire in both T-cell lines was reduced on the basis of usage of certain TCRBV gene families in comparison to paired control PBL. However, the T-lymphocyte repertoire of GITL propagated from the second biopsy was more extensive when compared to the repertoire of GITL propagated from the first biopsy. These results demonstrate that mH antigens could play a critical role in renal allograft rejection in HLA-identical siblings and that they are expressed on PTEC. Furthermore the T-cell response against the renal allograft seems to be mediated initially by T cells with a restricted TCRBV gene family usage. As the rejection process progresses, the diversity of the T lymphocytes which accumulate into the renal allograft increases.

7.1 INTRODUCTION

The immune response against foreign tissues can be directed against alloantigenic differences between donor and recipient, encoded by genes of the major histocompatibility complex (MHC, HLA in man). However, when MHC antigens are identical, as in HLA identical-siblings, graft rejection may still occur and will by definition be directed against minor histocompatibility antigens (mH).[1-5] Historically, mH loci have been viewed as independently segregating genetic loci that are scattered through the genome.[6] The existence of mH antigens has been conclusively demonstrated both in humans and mice, and their chromosomal localization has been determined.[7-8]

MHC class I restricted CD4$^-$CD8$^+$ cytotoxic T lymphocytes (CTL) are commonly accepted as being important effectors of immune responses against minor H antigens. However, CD4$^+$CD8$^-$ MHC class II restricted T helper cells may be required for the induction phase of the immune response.[9-11]

Since in biopsies from rejecting renal allografts, graft-infiltrating T lymphocytes (GITL) can be found in close association with renal tubuli often leading to tubular destruction, expression of mH antigens on tubular cells is of potential importance. Indeed, it has been shown[12] that CTL defined mH antigens are present on proximal tubular epithelial cells (PTEC). In addition, we have previously shown that GITL may be directly cytotoxic against PTEC.[13-15]

In this study we report on the isolation of two GITL cell lines isolated from two biopsies of the same patient suffering from two successive rejection episodes. The patient had received a kidney from his HLA-identical brother. Both cell lines propagated from GITL were highly cytotoxic against both PTEC and PHA stimulated peripheral blood lymphocytes (PBL) of donor origin. No effect on cytotoxicity could be seen upon treatment of PTEC with 200 U/ml of interferon

(IFN) gamma for 72 hours. Inhibition of cytotoxicity could be established with anti-CD3, anti-CD8, anti-CD18 and anti-MHC class I monoclonal antibodies (MoAb), both on PHA blasts and PTEC as target cells. Both GITL cell lines displayed a polyclonal TCRBV gene repertoire on the basis of TCRBV gene usage. The T-cell receptor repertoire of the GITL cell line isolated from the second biopsy was more diverse than GITL isolated from the first biopsy. This observation is in concert with the hypothesis that initially the immune response against the allograft is mediated by only a few T-cell clones. As the rejection process advances, more cells will migrate and accumulate into the graft, leading to a polyclonal inflammatory process.

This study shows that mH antigens, not previously described on PTEC, are recognized by GITL. We put forward the hypothesis that they could play a critical role in the rejection process of an HLA identical renal transplant from a living related donor.

7.2 MATERIALS AND METHODS

CASE REPORT

A 53 year old man received an HLA identical kidney from his 45 year old brother on March 16, 1992. He was diagnosed to have renal insufficiency of unknown origin in 1989 when he presented himself with gout. Hemodialysis was started in January 1992. There was an uneventful course immediate post-operation and his serum creatinine stabilized around 85 micromol/l from day 5 on, corresponding to a creatinine clearance of 91 ml/min. The patient received prednisone (starting dose 110 mg rapidly tapered off to 25 mg daily) and azathioprine (1.5 mg/kg) as maintenance immunosuppression. The level of his serum creatinine increased on post-operation day 17 and there was clear evidence for sodium retention and development of fever (temperature 39.2°C). A sonogram of the kidney showed no signs of post-renal obstruction and an infection causing the fever could not be identified. A renal biopsy containing only four glomeruli showed no signs of rejection. Since there was further deterioration of renal function on day 19 (serum creatinine 373 micromol/l) a three day course of intravenous methylprednisolone (1 gram daily) was started. The temperature normalized and the serum creatinine decreased somewhat to 357 micromol/l on day 22. However, in the subsequent days there was no further improvement in renal function and a second biopsy was performed on day 24.

The tissue specimen contained 9 glomeruli with endothelial swelling and an influx of inflammatory cells present in the capillary loops. There were also a few inflammatory cells present in the peritubular capillaries, but there was not enough infiltrate to make the diagnosis "interstitial rejection." The glomerular abnormalities were felt to be compatible with the diagnosis "transplant glomerulopathy."

A ten day course with rabbit-antithymocyte globulin (RATG) was started and the patient was converted from azathioprine to cyclosporin (starting dose 10 mg/kg) maintenance therapy. His serum creatinine came down to 125 micromol/l corresponding with a creatinine clearance of 60 ml/min. With this regimen there were no further rejection episodes and his renal function has remained stable.

METHODS FOR CELL CULTURE PROCEDURES

Both methods for culturing PTEC and graft infiltrating T lymphocyte (GITL) have been extensively described elsewhere (see Miltenburg et al.[14]). Briefly, GITL were cultured in Iscove's modified Dulbecco's medium (IMDM) with 10% fetal calf serum (FCS) and 5% T-cell growth factor (TCGF). Isolated cell lines were thereafter stimulated weekly using irradiated (3000 rad) peripheral blood mononuclear cells (PBMC) and OKT3 ascites. Biopsies were only done on clinical grounds. For this investigation one extra puncture (18 gauge Biopty[R]-system, Sweden) was performed during the biopsy procedure under echographic guidance. This study was approved by the Medical Ethics Committee of the University Hospital Leiden, and informed consent was obtained from the patient.

Donor PBL were isolated by a Ficoll-Hypaque gradient and stimulated with PHA (0.1 µg/ml; Sigma, St. Louis, MO, U.S.A.) in IMDM supplemented with 10% FCS and 5% TCGF. PTEC were cultured in a specific serum free medium following the protocol of Detrisac et al.[16]

CHARACTERIZATION OF PTEC AND PHENOTYPING OF GITL CELL LINES

PTEC were characterized by binding of a monoclonal antibody (MoAb) directed against anti-epithelial membrane antigen (EMA, Dakes, Glostrup, Denmark) and two other MoAbs (1071 and 1072) directed against adenosine deaminase binding protein (kindly provided by Dr. Dinjens, University Hospital, Maastricht, The Netherlands). Phenotyping of GITL lines was performed using FACS analysis. Staining was done by a two steps immunofluorescense technique using MoAbs directed against CD3 (OKT3), CD4 (OKT4), CD8 (OKT8) and TCR α/β (WT31), (all from ATCC, Rockville, MD, U.S.A.) as first antibody followed by a goat anti-mouse FITC conjugated IgG (Becton and Dickinson).

CYTOTOXICITY ASSAYS

Cytotoxicity was measured using a standard ^{51}Cr release assay. Briefly, target cells were labeled with 100 µCi of ^{51}Cr for 1 hour at 37°C, 5% CO_2. After washing twice, 5.10^3 labeled cells were put in each well of a 96 well plate (U bottom Costar, Cambridge, MA, U.S.A.) containing 4 different concentrations of effector cells (total volume 200 µl).

The plate was centrifuged (1200 rpm, 5 min) and incubated for 4 hours at 37°C, 5% CO_2. Thereafter the plate was centrifuged again and 100 μl of each well was harvested and counted in a gamma counter. In each experiment, for each target a medium control and a Triton X-100 control was included. Specific ^{51}Cr release was calculated by the formula:

$$\% \text{ specific release} = \frac{\text{CPM sample - CPM medium x } 100\%}{\text{CPM Triton X-100 - CPM medium}}$$

Blocking experiments were performed with anti-HLA class II (B8.11,2 a gift from Dr. M. Giphart, Department of Immunohematology and Bloodbank, University Hospital Leiden, The Netherlands), anti-HLA class I (W6/32), anti-CD3 (OKT3), anti-CD4 (OKT4), anti-CD8 (OKT8) and anti-CD18 (IB4) (all from ATCC Rockville, MD, U.S.A.) in an ascites dilution of 1:100. Antibodies were present during the assay.

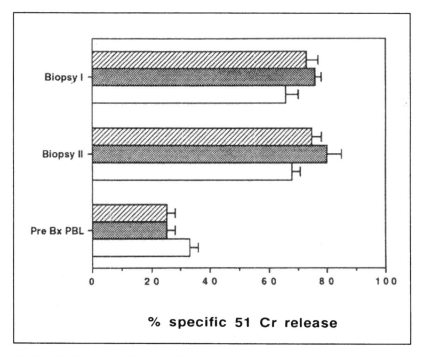

Fig. 7.1. T cells isolated from two biopsies and from PBL were tested in a standard ^{51}Cr release assay, using PTEC (hatched bars), PTEC incubated for 72 hours with 200 U/ml of IFN gamma (stippled bars) and PHA stimulated PBL (open bars) all of donor origin as target cells. An effector/target (E/T) ratio of 50 was used. Results are expressed as % specific ^{51}Cr release ± SD.

RNA Isolation, PCR Amplification
and Characterization of Amplified Products

Total RNA was isolated from approximately 10^7 T cells by extraction with RNAzol (Cinna/Biotecx Laboratories Inc, Houston, TX, U.S.A.). 5 µg of total RNA was converted into first strand cDNA using oligo dT primers according to the manufacturer's instructions (Promega Corporation, Madison, WI, U.S.A.). PCR amplification and Southern blot analysis were essentially the same as previously described (Lambert et al.;[17] Struyk et al.[37]).

7.3 RESULTS

Two GITL cell lines were isolated from the same patient suffering from two successive rejection episodes. These lines were highly cyto-

Table 7.1. Phenotyping of PBL and two GITL lines from two successive biopsies

line from	anti-CD3	anti-CD4	anti-CD8	anti-TCR α/β
biopsy I	97[a]	34	69	100
biopsy II	95	40	65	98
PBL	100	58	39	99

[a]: % positive cells

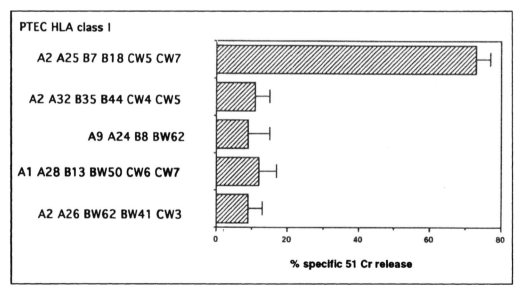

Fig. 7.2. GITL isolated from the second biopsy were tested for cytotoxicity on donor PTEC (top bar) and other HLA typed PTEC lines. Cytotoxicity was tested at an E/T ratio of 50. Results are expressed as % specific ^{51}Cr release ± SD.

toxic against cultured PTEC and PHA stimulated PBL both of donor origin. In addition PBL isolated at the time of the second rejection displayed cytotoxicity against both donor target cells, although to a lesser extent than the two GITL lines. Anti-donor reactivity is therefore not exclusively located in the graft (Fig. 7.1).

PBL isolated before transplantation were not cytotoxic against PTEC or PHA blasts. Treatment of PTEC with 200 U/ml of IFN gamma for 72 hours, a condition known to upregulate MHC class I and to induce MHC class II expression, had no effect on PTEC lysis by the GITL cell lines. With FACS analysis relatively more CD4⁻CD8⁺ T cells were found in both T-cell lines in comparison to paired PBL (Table 7.1).

Since GITL were cultured in the presence of TCGF, cytotoxicity theoretically could be due to lymphokine activated killer cell (LAK) activity. Therefore the specificity of PTEC lysis by these GITL cell lines was investigated. Both GITL cell lines were cytotoxic in a donor specific fashion as could be demonstrated by using third party PTEC lines as target cells in a standard ^{51}Cr release assay. Cytotoxicity was therefore due to specific recognition of target molecules on PTEC (Fig. 7.2). Target cell lysis could be inhibited using MoAb against

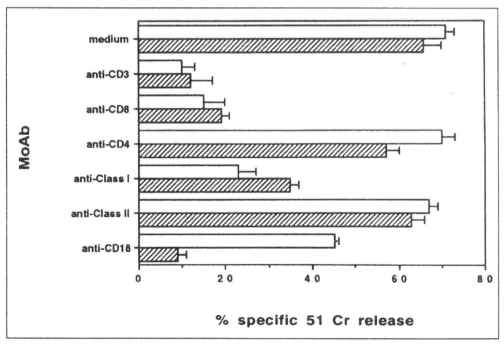

Fig. 7.3. Inhibition of lysis of PTEC (hatched bars) and PHA blasts (open bars) with MoAb. Antibodies were used in a dilution of 1:50 from ascites and were present during the assay. Cytotoxicity was measured at an E/T ratio of 50. Results are expressed as % specific ^{51}Cr release ± SD.

anti-CD3, anti-CD8, anti-MHC class I and anti-CD18 (Fig. 7.3). Consequently, cytotoxicity is T cell mediated and MHC class I restricted. Inhibition by anti-CD18 MoAb with PTEC as targets was stronger than with PHA blasts. The LFA-1/ICAM-1 adhesion pathway seems to be the major adhesion pathway between PTEC and T lymphocytes, whereas in the T-T cell interaction other adhesion pathways seem to have more relevance.

In order to investigate how the mH antigens were inherited, a family study was performed using PBL from several members of the patient's family (Fig. 7.4). Cytoxicity of GITL against PBL could be demonstrated on PBL carrying the HLA haplotype A25, B18, CW7. However not all PBL targets carrying this haplotype were recognized by the GITL. No specific MHC class I restriction element was observed.

It has been suggested that oligoclonality or polyclonality of the T cell response against the graft may depend on the degree of HLA matching and the time interval between transplantation and rejection.[18,19] GITL lines were isolated from two successive rejection episodes, one week and two weeks after transplantation respectively. To investigate

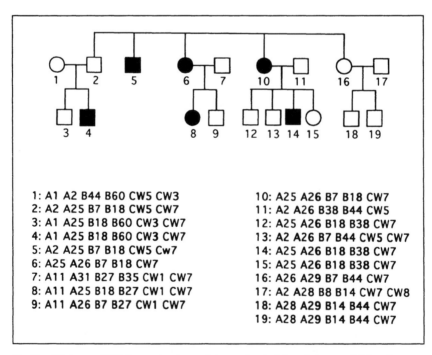

1: A1 A2 B44 B60 CW5 CW3

2: A2 A25 B7 B18 CW5 CW7

3: A1 A25 B18 B60 CW3 CW7

4: A1 A25 B18 B60 CW3 CW7

5: A2 A25 B7 B18 CW5 Cw7

6: A25 A26 B7 B18 CW7

7: A11 A31 B27 B35 CW1 CW7

8: A11 A25 B18 B27 CW1 CW7

9: A11 A26 B7 B27 CW1 CW7

10: A25 A26 B7 B18 CW7

11: A2 A26 B38 B44 CW5

12: A25 A26 B18 B38 CW7

13: A2 A26 B7 B44 CW5 CW7

14: A25 A26 B18 B38 CW7

15: A25 A26 B18 B38 CW7

16: A26 A29 B7 B44 CW7

17: A2 A28 B8 B14 CW7 CW8

18: A28 A29 B14 B44 CW7

19: A28 A29 B14 B44 CW7

Fig. 7.4. HLA typed PBL from members of the patient's (2) and donor's (5) family were tested for cytotoxicity using GITL isolated from the second biopsy as effector cells. Cytotoxicity was measured at four different E/T ratios for each target. Males (squares) and female (circles) were included and susceptibility to lysis (closed symbols) are depicted.

the nature of the T-cell receptor repertoire of T cell lines propagated from both biopsies, the TCRBV gene usage of T cells of each cell line was determined using a semi quantitative PCR technique. In addition, the TCRBV gene usage of PBL isolated at the time of the second rejection and cultured in a similar fashion as both GITL cell lines, was studied in parallel. Dominance of certain TCRBV gene usage could be seen in both cell lines in comparison to control PBL. (Fig. 7.5). Furthermore the second cell line showed a more extensive TCRBV repertoire compared to the first GITL derived cell line, suggesting a more polyclonal infiltration of T lymphocytes as the rejection process advances.

7.4 DISCUSSION

It is now well established that non-MHC encoded mH alloantigenic differences between donor and recipient may cause graft rejection. Most of these studies have been performed in murine models of allograft rejection.[2,4,20-23] In such models it is possible to study the effect of single mH antigen differences on graft survival by using congenic strain combinations.[10,11,20,21] In humans however it is impossible to asses the in vivo importance of single mH antigens in transplantation. The relevance of mH antigens has been shown in many studies by the occurrence of acute or chronic graft-versus-host disease (GvHD) after HLA identical bone marrow transplantation.[24-26] Minor H

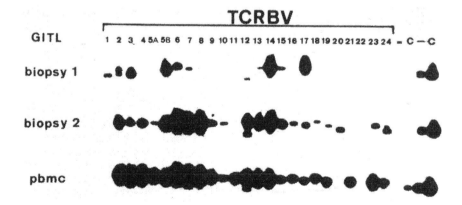

Fig. 7.5. GITL from both biopsies were analyzed for TCRBV gene usage by semiquantitative PCR as described previously (Lambert et al.;[17] Struyk et al.[37]). PBLs isolated at the time of the second rejection and cultured in a similar fashion were analyzed in parallel. A PCR reaction mixture without cDNA template was used in every reaction as negative control. In addition a PCR reaction using a TCRBC specific primer was run in parallel in order to correct for differences in the amount of cDNA between the samples. This positive control was put in three dilutions on the agarose gel.

antigens are present on cultured keratinocytes and can be recognized by mH specific CTL clones.[27] This is compatible with the skin lesions found in GvHD disease.[28,29]

In solid organ transplantation, like in renal transplantation, the actual risk of graft rejection is about 30% at 10 to 15 years post transplantation when the donor is an HLA identical sibling.[30,31] This suggests that at least some mH antigens must be expressed on renal tissues. Moreover it has been shown recently that cultured PTEC express CTL defined mH antigens.[12]

During interstitial renal allograft rejection GITL can be found in close association with renal tubuli and can cause tubular destruction. Previously we have demonstrated that isolated GITL from such kidneys were directly cytotoxic against cultured PTEC.[13-15] In the present study we report on the isolation and cytotoxicity against targets of donor origin, of two GITL lines from a patient receiving an HLA identical kidney from his brother. Although histologically there were no signs of rejection in the first biopsy and only a few inflammatory cells could be detected in the second biopsy, the patient responded favorably to anti-rejection therapy. Previously we showed that the outgrowth of GITL from biopsies correlated to the finding of rejection.[13] Thus culturing GITL from renal biopsies may give a better impression of the ongoing rejection process. Both GITL lines were highly cytotoxic against PTEC and PHA stimulated PBL both of donor origin. Cytotoxicity was not due to LAK activity since there was a specific recognition of certain HLA typed targets as demonstrated by using a panel of HLA typed PTEC (Fig. 7.2). Moreover it seemed that the cytotoxicity was related to a defined HLA haplotype when PBL from members of the patient's family were tested in a cytotoxicity assay. Cytotoxicity was related to the haplotype HLA-A25, B18, CW7. Susceptibility to lysis was inherited independently from this haplotype as would be expected from mH antigens.

Two other studies (Pfeffer et al.[32,33]) have shown that minor antigens can play a role in renal allograft rejection. In these studies it was suggested that the male H-Y minor antigen was of importance for the rejection episode, although the influence of other mH antigens could not be assessed. In this study however the male H-Y mH antigen was not involved in the rejection process since both patient and donor are of the same sex. In addition our study differs from previous reports in the way the effector cells were isolated. GITL were isolated directly from the site of inflammation and tested against renal cells, whereas PBL were used by others both as effector and target cells. Furthermore, using the patient's PBL as effector cells, cytotoxicity against donor PBL in the previous reports could only be assessed after in vitro restimulation with donor PBL. Our results however were obtained without restimulation with donor PBL. Although PBL isolated at the time of the second rejection displayed cytotoxicity against PTEC, a clear enrichment of cytotoxicity was observed in the GITL cell lines. Therefore specific infiltration of T lymphocytes reactive with mH antigens expressed on renal tissue may have occurred. Expression of these mH antigens however, was not tissue-specific since donor PHA blasts were lysed to the same extent.

The observed cytotoxicity of both GITL cell lines was T cell mediated and HLA-class I restricted as demonstrated by inhibition with MoAb against CD3, CD8 and MHC class I. Furthermore the interaction of GITL with PTEC was almost completely dependent on the LFA-1/ICAM-1 adhesion pathway. This is compatible with reports of Suranyi et al.,[34] who also showed inhibition of lysis of PTEC using anti-LFA-1 or anti-ICAM-1 antibodies. In contrast to PTEC lysis, inhibition of lysis of PHA blasts was less pronounced using anti-CD18 antibodies. This may be explained by the usage of other adhesion pathways in T-T cell interaction. Several reports have suggested that the CD2/LFA3 interaction may be used as adhesion pathway in T-T cell interaction.[35,36]

The usage of certain TCRBV gene families may depend on the differences in HLA between donor and recipient.[18,19] In a previous study (Yard et al.[13]) we could not correlate TCRBV dominance of GITL cell lines with HLA mismatches. Furthermore polyclonality of some GITL cell lines, isolated from biopsies one week after transplantation, could be demonstrated. However GITL were isolated from biopsies of patients receiving a kidney from a cadaveric donor and the TCRBV repertoire of GITL was analyzed only at one time after transplantation. In the present study the two GITL cell lines, isolated with a one week time interval, showed a limited TCRBV gene usage in comparison to the PBL control. GITL isolated from the second biopsy displayed more polyclonality than the GITL isolated from the first biopsy. This is compatible with the hypothesis that initially the immune response against the graft is mediated by a limited number of different T cell clones. As the rejection process advances more cells will be recruited to the graft, leading to a polyclonal infiltration.

Taken together these results clearly show that GITL isolated from biopsies from a patient grafted with an HLA identical kidney from his brother, are cytotoxic against cultured PTEC from the donor. Since during rejection GITL are found in close association with renal tubuli and tubuli seem to be destroyed by infiltrating T lymphocytes, expression of mH antigens on PTEC may be crucial in the effector phase of the rejection process. This study confirms and extends previous reports on the relevance of mH antigens and reports on the expression of unidentified mH antigens in renal allograft rejection in HLA-identical siblings.

ACKNOWLEDGEMENTS

This research was supported by the Dutch Kidney Foundation (Grant no. C 88 812) and by the J.A. Cohen Institute for Radiopathology and Radiation Protection (IRS).

REFERENCES

1. Snell GD, Dausset J, Nathenson S. In: Histocompatibility. Harcourt Brace Jovanovich (publ.). Academic Press New York, San Francisco, San Diego, London.

2. Loveland B, Simpson E. The non MHC transplantation antigens: Neither weak nor minor. Immunol Today 1986; 7:223-29.

3. Auchincloss H, Sachs DH. Transplantation and graft rejection. In: Paul WE, ed. Fundamental Immunology. New York: Raven, 1989:889-922.

4. Perreault C, Décary F, Brochu S et al. Minor histocompatibility antigens. Blood 1990: 76:1269-80.

5. Roopenian DC. 1992. What are minor histocompatibility loci? A new look at an old question. Immunol Today 1992; 13:7-10.

6. Motta R, Moutier R, Hall-Panenko O. Minor histocompatibility genes important in lethal graft-versus-host reaction (GVHR): Chromosomal assignment of five genes using ten chromosomal markers. Transplant Proc 1981; 13:1207-14.

7. Goulmy E, Gratema WJ, Blokland E et al. A minor transplantation antigen detected by MHC-restricted cytotoxic T lymphocytes during graft-versus-host disease. Nature 1983; 302:159-61.

8. Irle C, Beatty PG, Mickelson E et al. Alloreactive T cell responses between HLA-identical siblings. Detection of anti-minor histocompatibility T cell clones induced in vivo. Transplantation 1985; 40:329-33.

9. Roopenian DC, Anderson PS. Transplantation 1988; 46:899-904.

10. Roopenian DC, Widmer MB, Orosz CG et al. Responses against single minor histocompatibility antigens. I. Functional and immunogenetic analysis of cloned cytolytic T cells. J Immunol 1983; 131:2135-40.

11. Roopenian DC, Orosz CG, Bach FH. Responses against single minor histocompatibility antigens. II. Analysis of cloned helper T cells. J Immunol 1984; 132:1080-84.

12. De Bueger M, Bakker A, van Rood JJ et al. Tissue distribution of human minor histocompatibility antigens. Ubiquitous versus restricted tissue distribution indicates heterogeneity among human CTL defined non-MHC antigens. J Immunol 1992; 149:1788-94.

13. Yard BA, Kooymans-Couthino M, Reterink T et al. T cell lines isolated from rejecting renal allografts: Analysis of outgrowth, donor- and tissue specificity and T cell receptor Vβ gene usage. Kidney Int 1993; 43:133-38.

14. Miltenburg AMM, Paape ME, Daha MR et al. Donor-specific lysis of human kidney proximal tubular epithelial cells by renal allograft-infiltrated lymphocytes. Transplantation 1989; 48:296-302.

15. Van der Woude FJ, Daha MR, Miltenburg AMM et al. Renal allograft-infiltrated lymphocytes and proximal tubular cells: Further analysis of donor-specific lysis. Human Immunol 1990; 28:186-92.

16. Detrisac JC, Sens MA, Garvin AJ et al. Tissue culture of human kidney epithelial cells of proximal origin. Kidney Int 1984; 25:383-90.

17. Lambert M, van Eggermond M, Mascart F et al. TCR Vα and Vβ gene segment usage in T cell subcultures derived from a type III bare lymphocyte patient deficient in MHC class II expression. Developmental Immunol 1992; 2:227-36.

18. Hand SL, Hall BL, Finn OJ. T cell receptor Vβ gene usage in HLA-DR1-reactive human T cell populations. The predominance of Vβ8. Transplantation 1992; 54:357-67.

19. Miceli MC, Finn OJ. T cell receptor β-chain selection in human allograft rejection. J Immunol 1989; 142:81-86.

20. Wettstein PJ, Haughton G, Frelinger JA. H-2 effects on cell-cell interaction in the response to single non H-2 alloantigens. I. Donor H-2D region control of H-7.1 Immunogenicity and lack of restriction in vivo. J Exp Med 1977; 146:1346-55.

21. Wettstein PJ, Frelinger JA. H-2 effects on cell-cell interactions in the response to single non H-2 alloantigens. II. H-2D region control of H-7.1 specific stimulator function in mixed lymphocyte culture and susceptibility to lysis by H-7.1 specific cytotoxic cells. J Exp Med 1977; 146:1356-66.

22. Ando KI, Isobe KI, Hasegawa T et al. Genetic and stimulator cell requirements for generation and activation of minor histocompatibility antigen specific memory cytotoxic T lymphocyte precursors. Immunology 1988; 64:661-67.

23. Ando K, Nakashima I, Nagase F et al. Induction and characterization of minor histocompatibility antigens. Specific primary cytotoxic T lymphocyte responses in vitro. J Immunol 1988; 140:723-29.

24. Perreault C, Gyger M, Boileau J et al. Acute graft-versus-host disease after allogeneic bone marrow transplantation. Can Med Assoc J 1983; 129:969-74.

25. Storb R, Deeg HJ, Pepe M et al. Graft-versus-host disease prevention by methotrexate combined with cyclosporine compared to methotrexate alone in long-term follow-up of a controlled trial. Br J Heamatol 1989; 72:567-72.

26. Storb R, Deeg HJ, Appelbaum F et al. Methotraxate and cyclosporine versus cyclosporine alone for prophylaxis of graft versus-host-disease in patients given HLA-identical marrow grafts for leukemia: Long-term follow-up of a controlled trial. Blood 1989; 73:1729-34.

27. De Bueger M, Bakker A, van Rood JJ et al. Minor histocompatibility antigens, defined by graft-vs-host disease-derived cytotoxic T lymphocytes, show variable expression on human skin cells. Eur J Immunol 1991; 21:2839-44.

28. Piquet PF, Grau GE, Allet B et al. Tumor necrosis factor/cachectin is an effector of skin and gut lesions of the acute phase of graft vs host disease. J. Exp. Med. 1987; 166:1280-89.

29. Lampert IA, Janossy G, Suiters AJ et al. Immunological analysis of the skin in graft versus host disease. Clin Exp Immunol 1982; 50:123-31.
30. Albrechtsen D, Moen T, Flatmark et al. Influence of HLA-A,B,C,D and DR matching in renal transplantation. Transpl Proc 1981; 13:924-29.
31. Busson M, Hors J, Prevost P et al. Importance of HLA-A,B and -DR matching in presensitized kidney transplant recipients. Clin Transpl 1988; 199-202.
32. Pfeffer PF, Gabrielsen TS, Ahonen J et al. Cytotoxic cells recognizing minor histocompatibility antigens in patients rejecting HLA-identical grafts. Transpl Proc 1983; 15:1821-22.
33. Pfeffer PF, Thorsby. HLA-restricted cytotoxicity against male-specific (H-Y) antigen after acute rejection of an HLA-identical sibling kidney. Transplantation 1982; 33:52-56.
34. Suranyi MG, Bishop A, Clayberger C et al. Lymphocyte adhesion molecules in T cell-mediated lysis of human kidney cells. Kidney Int 1991; 39:312-19.
35. Mentzer SJ, Smith BR, Barbosa JA et al. CTL adhesion and antigen recognition are discrete steps in the human CTL-target cell interaction. J Immunol 1987; 138:1325-30.
36. Shaw S, Ginther Luce GE, Quinones R et al. Two antigen-independent adhesion pathways used by human cytotoxic T-cell clones. Nature 1986; 323:262-64.
37. Struyk L, Kurnick JT, Hawes GE et al. T-cell receptor V-gene usage in synovial fluid lymphocytes of patients with chronic arthritis. Hum Immunol 1993; 37:237-51.

CHAPTER 8

CONCLUDING REMARKS

Peter J. van den Elsen

Allorecognition can be considered in many ways as recognition of complexes of (allo) MHC and (allo) peptide. The question remains as to whether the T-cell response against these complexes of MHC and peptide expressed on the cell surface of an allograft displays a diverse character on the basis of T-cell receptor diversity or whether there is indeed selection at the level of the T-cell receptor by antigen-specific T cells.

Considering models of T-cell recognition, there is mounting evidence to support the notion that MHC class II associated T-cell responses against defined peptide antigens and MHC class II alleles in general might be heterogeneous with respect to T-cell receptor V-gene usage and/or amino acid composition of the CDR3.[1-4] This could be a reflection of the flexibility in the presentation of antigenic peptides by MHC class II antigens which might be related to the MHC class II peptide-binding site that is open at both ends. Brown et al.[5] have shown that as a result of the open-ended class II MHC peptide-binding groove, peptides can be bound in an extended conformation projecting out of both ends.[5] This may offer a more flexible overall conformation of the MHC class II-peptide complex.

The peptide elution studies have revealed the presence of peptides of 14-24 amino acids in length being associated with the peptide-binding groove of class II MHC molecules.[6-8] These MHC class II-associated peptides are longer than those found to be associated with MHC class I molecules. A longer peptide may offer more variability in the availability of amino acids within the bound peptide which serve as contact residues for the CDR-loops of the αβ T-cell receptor. In this respect, Nanda et al.[9] have shown that even in a relative small multideterminant peptide, each determinant is recognized by a different TCRBV gene segment.[9] Furthermore, naturally processed epitopes that are available may further restrict the responding repertoire, as there seems to be some individual-specific variation

The Human T-Cell Receptor Repertoire and Transplantation, edited by Peter J. van den Elsen. © 1995 R.G. Landes Company.

in epitope processing and presentation.[10] In the MHC class II system, epitopes defined as being promiscuous are also frequently described (see chapter 1). These promiscuous peptides are able to bind to different MHC class II alleles using different anchor residues comprised within the peptide. As a result different peptide side chains become available for interaction with the T-cell receptor allowing for a broader range of possible T-cell receptor capable of recognizing the epitope within one individual.[11]

Considering the above raised points, the diversity of the T-cell receptor repertoire used in the recognition of peptide-antigens presented by class II MHC molecules might prove to be diverse as a result of the flexibility offered by the MHC class II molecules in the presentation of the antigenic peptide for T-cell receptor interaction. It should be noted however, that there is evidence to suggest that clonal selection for T cells recognizing antigenic peptides presented by class II MHC molecules in vivo is evident. This has been demonstrated in studies to the nature of the immune-response in autoimmune and infectious diseases.[12-14] These observations reveal the existence of important in vivo selection mechanisms for T-cell receptor specificity, which merits further investigation.

As discussed in chapter 1, the peptides presented by class I MHC molecules are generally short (9 to 11 amino acids) which contrasts with what has been observed for peptides presented by class II MHC molecules (see chapter 1). Furthermore, MHC class I antigen presentation has demonstrated very strict properties in regard to the nature of the peptides that are bound to the groove of the MHC class I molecule offering less flexibility in the way the peptide-antigens are presented by the class I MHC molecules to the T-cell receptor.

Evidence is accumulating in the literature that the T-cell response against these MHC class I-peptide complexes is very restricted. Interindividual conservation of T-cell receptor β-chains used by the αβ T-cell receptor for the recognition of a defined peptide in the context of a given MHC class I allele has been reported.[15-18] This has clearly been demonstrated in the influenza virus A matrix peptide model where a conservation in the usage of the TCRBV17 V-gene among multiple individuals sharing the HLA-A*0201 allele was noted.[15,17] In a similar fashion, we recently demonstrated that T-cell reactivity against the minor histocompatibility antigen HA-1 in the context of HLA-A*0201 was noted for the sharing of the TCRBV6S9 gene segment.[18] This cellular encoded antigen plays a crucial role in the outcome of HLA-identical bone marrow transplantation.

On the basis of the above discussed points regarding T-cell recognition of a given peptide-antigen presented by defined class II or class I MHC alleles, it might be expected that in transplantation for MHC class I mediated responses against a complex of a given allo-peptide and MHC allele, the T-cell receptor V-gene usage might be restricted.

Since the allo-MHC molecules on the graft are capable of presenting pools of peptides to T cells, it should be taken into account that the T-cell repertoire of the host, which is shaped on the basis of recognizing the myriad of different peptides presented by autologous MHC class I alleles, is able to respond to differences in these pools of peptides presented by the MHC-molecules expressed on the cell surface of the allograft. As a consequence, the alloresponse might be more diverse than expected because the pool of peptides exhibits allele and individual-specific differences in the nature of the presented peptides. This recognition therefore can be regarded as a class I MHC-mediated immune response against a variety of specific complexes of MHC and peptide. However, assuming the existence of immunodominant peptide-epitopes that are being presented to the host immune system, clonal dominance of the responding T cells might be expected.

In the case of HLA-identical genetically related transplantations, like as occurring in monozygotic twins or in HLA-identical family transplantations, only minor differences might exist between the myriad of peptides presented by the HLA molecules of the recipient and the donor. As a consequence the immune repertoire of the host responding to the differences in the presented peptide pool might exhibit features of restriction as is found in systems of viral and cellular peptides presented by defined class I MHC alleles. Only in those cases where it is possible to define specific immune responses against minor differences between the host and the recipient, it might prove to be useful to design novel immunoregulatory reagents directed against the responding T-cell repertoire.

With respect to the class II mediated presentation of foreign peptides by self MHC class II molecules, on the basis of collective data in the literature on allorecognition and recognition of specific MHC-peptide complexes in autoimmune and infectious diseases it has been demonstrated that the T-cell receptor repertoire might be diverse of nature with exceptions where a clear dominant T-cell response is noted.

Therefore, if one considers the design of novel immunotherapeutic reagents aiming at interfering in T-cell recognition of these allo-MHC peptide complexes on the basis of T-cell receptor specificity, it should be taken into account that the preferred intervention against a restricted T-cell response might currently only be feasible in cases where the recipient and donor are highly related and share expression of the same HLA alleles. Furthermore, since the target peptide-antigens are unknown and might exhibit individual-specific expression patterns, such therapies have to be tailor-made for each transplant patient. For practical considerations therefore one could envision other approaches which are of a more general nature and could be aimed at the induction of tolerance against the MHC alleles expressed by the graft or at interfering in the cytokine dependent T-cell activation or adhesion pathways.

In conclusion, more knowledge is needed as to how the allo-antigen specific effector T-cell repertoire is generated in vivo because this might reveal highly selected T-cell receptor specificities which would be suitable as targets for immunotherapeutic interventions aimed at the downregulation of the allo-specific immune response.

REFERENCES

1. Quayle AJ, Wilson KB, Li SH et al. Peptide recognition, T cell receptor usage and HLA restriction elements of human heat-shock protein (hsp) 60 and mycobacterial 65-kDa hsp-reactive T cell clones from rheumatoid synovial fluid. Eur J Immunol. 1992; 22:1315-22.
2. Boitel B, Ermonval M, Panina-Bordignon P et al. Preferential Vβ gene usage and lack of junctional sequence conservation among human toxin-derived peptide: Evidence for a dominant role of a germ-line encoded V region in antigen/major histocompatibility complex recognition. J Exp Med. 1992; 175:765-77.
3. De Magistris MT, Di Tommaso A, Domenighini M et al. Interaction of the pertussis toxin peptide containing residues 30-42 with DR1 and the T-cell receptors of 12 human T-cell clones. Proc. Natl. Acad. Sci. USA 1992; 89:2990-94.
4. Hawes GE, Struyk L, Godthelp BC et al. Limited restriction in the αβ TCR-αβ V region usage of Ag-specific clones: recognition of myelin basic protein (amino acids 84-102) and *Mycobacterium bovis* 65-kDa heat shock protein (amino acids 3-13) by T cell clones established from peripheral blood mononuclear cells of monozygotic twins and HLA-identical individuals. J Immunol. 1995; 154:555-66.
5. Brown JH, Jardetzky TS, Gorga JC et al. Three-dimensional structure of the human class II histocompatibility antigen HLA-DR1. Nature 1993; 364:33-39.
6. Srinivasan M, Domanico SZ, Kaumaya PTP et al. Peptides of 23 residues or greater are required to stimulate a high affinity class-II restricted T cell response. Eur J Immunol. 1993; 23:1011-16
7. Brown LE, Jackson DC, Tribbick G et al. Extension of a minimal T cell determinant allows relaxation of the requirement for particular residues within the determinant. Int Immunol. 1991; 3:1307-13
8. Rammensee HG, Friede T and Stevanovic S. MHC ligands and peptide motifs: first listing. Immunogenetics 1995; 41:178-228.
9. Nanda NK, Arzoo KK and Sercarz EE. In a small multideterminant peptide, each determinant is recognized by a different Vβ gene segment. J Exp Med. 1992; 176:297-302.
10. Demotz S, Matricardi PM, Irle D et al. Processing of tetanus toxin by human antigen-presenting cells: evidence for donor and epitope-specific processing pathways. J Immunol. 1989, 143:3881-86
11. Wucherpfennig KW, Sette A, Southwood S et al. Structural requirements for binding of an immunodominant myelin basic protein peptide to DR2 isotypes and for its recognition by human T cell clones. J Exp Med. 1994; 179:279-90.

12. Vandevijver C, Mertens N, Van den Elsen P, Medear R, Raus J and Zhang J. Clonal expansion of myelin basic protein-reactive T cells in patients with multiple sclerosis: restricted T cell receptor V gene rearrangements and CDR3 sequence. Eur J Immunol. 1995, 25:958-968.

13. Struyk L, Hawes GE, Chatilla MK, Breedveld FC, Kurnick JT and Van den Elsen PJ. T cell receptors in rheumatoid arthritis. Arth & Rheum. 1995, in press.

14. Van Schooten WCA, Long KJ, Van der Stoep N et al. T cell receptor β-chain usage in the T cell recognition of *Mycobacterium leprae* antigens in one tuberculoid leprosy patient. Proc Natl Acad Sci. USA. 1992; 89:11244-48.

15. Lehner PJ, Wang ECY, Moss PAH et al. Human HLA-A0201-restricted cytotoxic T lymphocyte recognition of Influenza A is dominated by T cells bearing the Vβ17 gene segment. J Exp Med. 1995, 181:79-91.

16. Bowness P, Moss PAH, Rowland-Jones S et al. Conservation of T cell receptor usage by HLA B27-restricted influenza-specific cytotoxic T lymphocytes suggests a general pattern for antigen-specific major histocompatibility complex class I restricted responses. Eur J Immunol. 1993, 23:1417-21.

17. Moss PAH, Moots RJ, Rosenberg WMC et al. Extensive conservation of α and β chains of the human T-cell antigen receptor recognizing HLA-A2 and influenza A matrix peptide. Proc. Natl. Acad. Sci. USA 1991, 88;8987-90.

18. Goulmy E, Pool J, Van den Elsen PJ. Interindividual conservation of TCRBV regions by minor histocompatibility antigen-specific HLA-A*0201-restricted CTL clones. Blood 1995, in press.

INDEX

Page numbers in italics denote figures (F) or tables (T).

MEDICAL INTELLIGENCE UNIT

AVAILABLE AND UPCOMING TITLES

Made in the USA
Columbia, SC
18 June 2021